Special Issue
Included in subscription

Pediatric Neurosurgery (ISSN 1016–2291),
Vol. 16, No. 4–5 (1990–91)
Editor: F.J. Epstein, New York, N.Y.

The E. Bruce Hendrick Festschrift

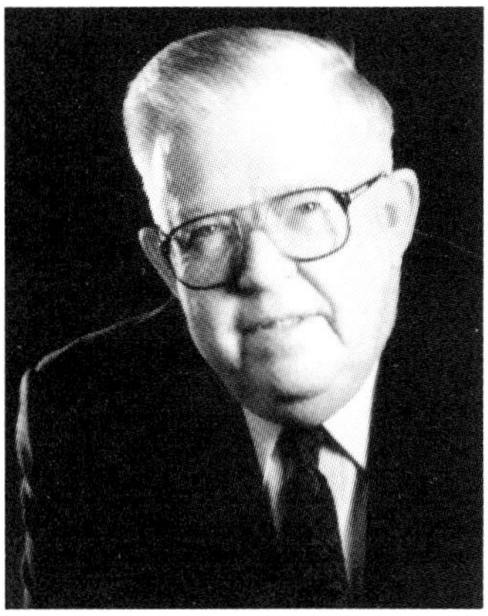

Editor:
R.P. Humphreys
Toronto

This special issue of *Pediatric Neurosurgery* is dedicated to E. Bruce Hendrick, Canada's first pediatric neurosurgeon and the first Editor-in-Chief of this journal, originally known as *Pediatric Neuroscience*. All former residents and fellows of The Hospital for Sick Children, Toronto, were invited to contribute a paper. Of the many manuscripts that were submitted, the editor selected those which focus on areas of special interest to E.B. Hendrick – hydrocephalus, spinal dysraphism, trauma, and tumor control. The result is a carefully edited *Festschrift* offering an excellent and up-to-date survey on these topics.

Contents

Fields of Interest

Neurology, Neurosurgery

The E. Bruce Hendrick Festschrift
'Pediatric Neurosurgery', Vol. 16, No. 4–5 (1990-91)
Editor: Humphreys, R.P. (Toronto)
96 p., 57 fig., 34 tab., soft cover, 1990-91
SFr. 52.– / DM 62.– / £ 22.60 / US$ 41.75
US$ price for USA, £ price for UK only (subject to change)
ISBN 3–8055–5580–6

KARGER

KI 92107

Stereotactic and Functional Neurosurgery

Official Journal of the World Society for Stereotactic and Functional Neurosurgery

Official Journal of the American Society for Stereotactic and Functional Neurosurgery

Founded 1938 as 'Confinia Neurologica' by E.A. Spiegel
Continued 1975–1988 as 'Applied Neurophysiology'

Publication data: 'Stereotactic and Functional Neurosurgery' is published 8 times annually. Volumes 58–59 with 4 issues each appear in 1992.

Subscription rates: Subscriptions run for a full calendar year. Prices are given per volume, surface postage included.

Personal subscription: SFr. 151.20, US$ 100.80. (Must be in the name of, billed to, and paid by an individual. Order must be marked 'personal subscription'.)

Institutional subscription: SFr. 216.–, US$ 144.00. (Regular rate.)

Members of the different Societies for Stereotactic and Functional Neurosurgery are requested to apply for appropriate discounts.

Airmail postage: SFr. 25.–, US$ 20.00. (Extra per volume.)

Microform subscription: SFr. 108.–, US$ 72.00. (Available exclusively to subscribers of the paper edition.)

Subscription orders: Orders can be placed at agencies, bookstores, directly with the Publisher S. Karger AG, P.O. Box, CH – 4009 Basel (Switzerland) or with any of the following distributors:

Deutschland:
S. Karger GmbH, Lörracher Strasse 16A
Postfach, D-W-7800 Freiburg

France: Librairie Luginbühl
36, bd de Latour-Maubourg, F – 75007 Paris

Great Britain, Ireland:
S. Karger Publishers, 11 Ravenscroft Road
Beckenham, Kent BR3 4TP

USA: S. Karger Publishers, Inc.
26 West Avon Road, P.O. Box 529
Farmington, CT 06085

India, Bangladesh, Sri Lanka:
S. Karger India Subscription Agency
B – 5/132 Safdarjung Enclave
New Delhi-110029

Japan: Katakura Libri, Inc.
36-9 Hongo 3-chome,
Bunkyo-ku, Tokyo 113

Change of address: Both old and new address should be stated and sent to the subscription source.

KARGER

Single issues and back volumes: Information on availability and prices can be obtained through the Publisher.

Bibliographic indices: This journal is regularly listed in bibliographic services, including *Current Contents®*.

Book Reviews: Books are accepted for review by special agreement.

Advertising: Correspondence and rate requests should be addressed to the Publisher.

Stereotact Funct Neurosurg
Printed in Switzerland by
Basler Zeitung AG, Basel

S. Karger AG,
Postfach, CH – 4009 Basel (Schweiz)

Erscheint anderthalbmonatlich;
pro Jahr 2 Bände zu 4 Heften

Submission: Only original papers written in English are considered and should be sent to:

Prof. Dr. Ph.L. Gildenberg
6560 Fannin Street, Suite 1530
Houston, TX 77030 (USA)

Manuscripts should be submitted in triplicate (with three sets of illustrations of which one is an original), typewritten double-spaced on one side of the paper, with a wide margin.

Conditions: All manuscripts are subjected to editorial review. Manuscripts are received with the explicit understanding that they are not under simultaneous consideration by any other publication. Submission of an article for publication implies the transfer of the copyright from the author to the publisher upon acceptance. Accepted papers become the permanent property of 'Stereotactic and Functional Neurosurgery' and may not be reproduced by any means, in whole or in part, without the written consent of the publisher. It is the author's responsibility to obtain permission to reproduce illustrations, tables, etc. from other publications.

Arrangement:

Title page: The first page of each paper should indicate the title (main title underlined), the authors' names, and the institute where the work was conducted. A short title for use as running head as well as the full address of the author to whom correspondence should be sent are also required.

Full address: The exact postal address complete with postal code of the senior author must be given at the bottom of the title page. Please also supply phone and fax numbers.

Key words: For indexing purposes, a list of 3–10 key words in English is essential.

Abstract: Each paper needs an abstract of up to 10 lines.

Small type: Paragraphs which can or must be set in smaller type (case histories, test methods, etc.) should be indicated with a 'p' (petit) in the margin on the left-hand side.

Footnotes: Avoid footnotes. When essential, they are numbered consecutively and typed at the foot of the appropriate page.

Tables and illustrations: Tables and illustrations (both numbered in Arabic numerals) should be prepared on separate sheets. Tables require a heading and figures a legend, also prepared on a separate sheet. For the reproduction of illustrations, only good drawings and original photographs can be accepted; negatives or photocopies cannot be used. When possible, group several illustrations on one block for reproduction (max. size 113 × 174 mm) or provide crop marks. On the back of each illustration, indicate its number, the author's name, and 'top'. Color illustrations are reproduced at the author's expense.

References: In the text identify references by Arabic numerals [in square brackets]. Material submitted for publication but not yet accepted should be noted as 'unpublished data' and not be included in the reference list. The list of references should include only those publications which are cited in the text. Do not alphabetize; number references in the order in which they are first mentioned in the text. The surnames of the authors followed by initials should be given. There should be no punctuation other than a comma to separate the authors. Cite all authors, 'et al' is not sufficient. Abbreviate journal names according to the Index Medicus system. (Also see International Committee of Medical Journal Editors: Uniform requirements for manuscripts submitted to biomedical journals. Br Med J 1988;296: 401–405.)

Examples

(a) Papers published in periodicals: Kauffman HF, van der Heide S, Beaumont F, Blok H, de Vries K: Class-specific antibody determination against *Aspergillus fumigatus* by means of the enzyme-linked immunosorbent assay. III. Comparative study: IgG, IgA, IgM ELISA titers, precipitating antibodies and IgE binding after fractionation of the antigen. Int Arch Allergy Appl Immunol 1986;80:300–306.

(b) Monographs: Matthews DE, Farewell VT: Using and Understanding Medical Statistics. Basel, Karger, 1985.

(c) Edited books: Hardy WD Jr, Essex M: FeLV-induced feline acquired immune deficiency syndrome: A model for human AIDS; in Klein E (ed): Acquired Immunodeficiency Syndrome. Prog Allergy. Basel, Karger, 1986, vol 37, pp 353–376.

Further details: Authors may consult our leaflet 'Rules for the Preparation of Manuscripts', available on request from the Publisher, S. Karger AG, P.O. Box, CH-4009 Basel (Switzerland).

Page charges: There is no page charge for papers of 8 or fewer printed pages (including tables, illustrations and references). Each additional complete or partial page is charged to the author at SFr. 225.– / US $ 150.00. The allotted size of a paper is equal to approx. 16 manuscript pages (including tables, illustrations and references).

Galley proofs: Unless indicated otherwise, galley proofs are sent to the first-named author and should be returned with the least possible delay. Alterations made in galley proofs, other than the correction of printer's errors, are charged to the author. No page proofs are supplied.

Reprints: Order forms and a price list are sent with the galley proofs. Orders submitted after the issue is printed are subject to considerably higher prices. Allow five weeks from date of publication for delivery of reprints.

KARGER

Proceedings of the
Meeting of the American Society for

Stereotactic and Functional Neurosurgery

Pittsburgh, Pa., June 16–19, 1991
Part I

Editors: *L. Dade Lunsford,* Pittsburgh, Pa.;
Philip L. Gildenberg, Houston, Tex.;
Patricia O. Franklin, Houston, Tex.

37 figures, 28 tables, 3 color plates, 1992

KARGER

S. Karger · Medical and Scientific Publishers
Basel · Freiburg · Paris · London · New York · New Delhi · Bangkok · Singapore · Tokyo · Sydney

Drug Dosage

The authors and the publisher have exerted every effort to ensure that drug selection and dosage set forth in this text are in accord with current recommendations and practice at the time of publication. However, in view of ongoing research, changes in government regulations, and the constant flow of information relating to drug therapy and drug reactions, the reader is urged to check the package insert for each drug for any change in indications and dosage and for added warnings and precautions. This is particularly important when the recommended agent is a new and/or infrequently employed drug.

Printed in Switzerland on acid-free paper by Basler Zeitung, Basel
ISBN 3-8055-5684-5

Contents

Computer and Technological Advances

Epilepsy

Proceedings of the Meeting of the American Society for Stereotactic and Functional Neurosurgery, Pittsburgh, Pa., June 16–19, 1991
Stereotact Funct Neurosurg 1992;58:1

Introduction

In June 1991, the American Society of Stereotactic and Functional Neurosurgery met in Pittsburgh, Pa., for its every 4 year meeting. The topics covered in detail at this meeting included surgery for epilepsy, movement disorders, spasticity and innovative management of a wide variety of cerebral mass lesions.

Stereotactic surgery has become a widely used technique, available at a number of institutions, increasingly a part of the mainstream field of neurological surgery. The use of intracranial guiding devices has facilitated diagnosis and treatment of a wide variety of brain pathologies, including neoplastic, vascular and degenerative disorders. In addition, members of the Society presented their experience in the management of movement disorders, epilepsy and spasticity, using techniques such as transplantation and neuroaugmentation.

Across the world, stereotactic instrumentation has combined with radiological imaging as well as therapeutic tools. The result has been an explosive growth in the field of stereotactic radiosurgery. An international meeting devoted to the topic of stereotactic radiosurgery was held immediately after the American Society of Stereotactic and Functional Neurosurgery meeting. Overall, the combined 5 day meeting attracted an international group of neurological surgeons, neurologists, radiologists, radiation oncologists and medical physicists.

Volume 58 and 59, 1992, describe the current state and status of many aspects of the fields of stereotactic surgery, functional surgery and radiosurgery.

I am indebted to the staff of the Continuing Medical Education Department of the University of Pittsburgh and to the staff of the Specialized Neurosurgical Center of the University of Pittsburgh Medical Center. Their efforts culminated in the success of these meetings.

L. Dade Lunsford, MD

Functional Neurosurgery and Tissue Transplantation

Proceedings of the Meeting of the American Society for Stereotactic and Functional Neurosurgery, Pittsburgh, Pa., June 16–19, 1991
Stereotact Funct Neurosurg 1992;58:3–13

Neurosurgical Treatment of Spasticity: Selective Posterior Rhizotomy and Intrathecal Baclofen

A. Leland Albright

Department of Neurosurgery, Children's Hospital, University of Pittsburgh School of Medicine, Pittsburgh, Pa., USA

Key Words. Spasticity · Rhizotomy · Intrathecal baclofen · Cerebral palsy

Abstract. The pathophysiology of spasticity and the history of posterior rhizotomies are reviewed. The rationale for selective posterior rhizotomies is that electrical stimulation identifies afferent posterior rootlets that terminate on relatively uninhibited alpha motoneurons; if these uninhibited rootlets are divided, spasticity can be alleviated without loss of other posterior root functions. Indications, technique, and results of selective posterior rhizotomies are presented. The use of continuous intrathecal baclofen (CITB) is summarized. CITB at doses of approximately 300 μg/day consistently reduces lower extremity spasticity and diminishes or alleviates muscle spasms in adults with spasticity of spinal origin. Single doses of intrathecal baclofen significantly decrease lower extremity muscle tone in children with cerebral palsy, and the effects can be maintained in these patients by CITB infusions which diminish muscle tone not only in the lower extremities, but in the upper extremities as well. CITB is best accomplished via an externally programmable pump that allows titration of the daily dose to attain the desired reduction in spasticity. Factors influencing the decision for rhizotomy or CITB are presented.

Pathophysiology of Spasticity

Spasticity – from the Greek word spastikos (to tug or draw) – is an abnormality of muscle tone in which there is increased resistance to passive muscle stretch. The muscle tone is regulated by the efferent output of alpha motoneurons. That efferent output is determined by competing impulses: (1) inhibitory impulses from basal ganglia, reticu-

1011–6125/92/0584–0003 $ 2.75/0

lar formation, and cerebellum that descend through the rubrospinal, reticulospinal, and vestibulospinal pathways, and (2) afferent excitatory impulses that arise from muscle spindles and travel in Ia fibers in the posterior root. Inhibitory and excitatory fibers terminate on interneurons which subsequently modulate alpha motoneurons. Diseases that damage the descending inhibitory pathways, either at their source (cerebral palsy, strokes) or along their descent (spinal cord trauma, multiple sclerosis), will cause spasticity.

Because many diseases can disrupt the inhibitory pathways, spasticity is a common disorder and has been treated – generally unsuccessfully – by neurosurgeons and neurologists. Surgical treatment has evolved through nonselective posterior and anterior rhizotomies, intrathecal phenol injections, myelotomies, and cerebellar stimulators to the current use of selective posterior rhizotomies. Medical treatment has evolved through oral anticonvulsants, alcohol neuromuscular blockers, baclofen, and dantrolene to the current use of intrathecal baclofen. As others have observed, the problems of spasticity are always the same, but the 'solutions' differ with each medical era.

Selective Posterior Rhizotomy (SPR)

SPR is an operation that has been evolving over the past century. The pathophysiologic basis for SPR lay in the neurophysiological studies of Sherrington [1] who in 1898 reported that cats with midbrain transsections developed extensor rigidity of all extremities and that, if posterior roots of an affected extremity were divided, the rigidity in that extremity was abolished. Foerster [2] in 1913, reported his treatment of 157 patients, including 88 children with spastic cerebral palsy, in whom he divided the entire posterior roots of L2–S1, leaving only the posterior root of L4. That procedure effectively alleviated lower extremity spasticity, but produced both ataxia and decubiti, and extensive nonselective posterior rhizotomies fell into disrepute.

Rhizotomies were modified by Gros et al. [3] to preserve 20% of each posterior root and by Sindou et al. [4] to disrupt the posterior root at the root entry zone, but Fasano [5] was probably the first to use physiological stimulation to determine which rootlets were to be divided. This author reported that a train of 50 stimuli applied for 1 s to a normal posterior lumbar root would cause a brief muscle contraction, followed rapidly by relaxation, but that if an identical stimulus were applied to the posterior root of a child with spastic cerebral palsy, 'abnormal' responses occurred: a tetanic muscle contraction that persisted throughout the stimulus or that might crescendo during the stimulus or persist even after the stimulus ceased. Fasano [5] reported that stimulation of posterior lumbar rootlets at the root entry zone gave variable findings – some normal and some abnormal. He divided the rootlets giving abnormal responses, generally 25–50% of the rootlets at each level from L2 to S1, and spasticity was effectively alleviated without loss of proprioception or sensation. The rationale for SPR is that stimulation identifies afferent rootlets that terminate on relatively uninhibited interneurons. Fasano's determination of a 'normal' response has not been verified by others; operative opportunities to stimulate normal lumbosacral nerve roots are limited. Laitenen et al. [6] treated 8 patients with lower and 1 patient with upper extremity spasticity with Fasano's procedure and replicated his results, but SPR remained relatively unutilized until it was modified and popularized by Peacock et al. [7].

The technique of Fasano [5] stimulated and divided lumbosacral posterior roots at the conus medullaris, where identification of nerve roots may be difficult, particularly the distinction between S1 and S2. Peacock [7] modified Fasano's procedure by performing the nerve stimulation near the root exit foramina, where nerves can be identified more easily, and he popularized the procedure. His technique and results have been replicated by others [8–10]. SPR has customarily been performed on the L2–S1 nerve rootlets (and S2 if there is spastic toe flexion). Recently, Lazareff et al. [11] reported that SPR of only the L4–S1 roots relieved lower extremity spasticity, including spasticity in the more proximally innervated iliopsoas and adductor muscles. Cervical SPR has been performed infrequently; it may decrease elbow and wrist flexor tone and improve range of motion, but the function is usually unaffected.

The two general goals of relieving spasticity by SPR, to facilitate patient care and to improve function, influence patient selection. Care is facilitated primarily for patients whose severe spasticity hampers sitting, dressing, and perineal care; SPR will also lessen their development of contractures. The function is facilitated primarily for children with spastic diplegia whose mild-to-moderate spasticity hampers their walking. SPR should be performed early, usually at the age of 3–7 years for these children; it can be performed to improve function in girls up to 13 years and in boys up to age 17 [7]. After that time gait patterns are difficult to change, and contractures are likely to be present. There are no age limitations for SPR to facilitate care. However, patients with moderate and severe untreated spasticity usually develop multiple contractures by their mid-20s, and the contractures minimize the benefits of SPR. Patients with unilateral spasticity may benefit from unilateral SPR; however, many such patients are quite functional because one side is normal; the goals of SPR must be carefully identified in these children.

Rhizotomies are performed under general anesthesia, without neuromuscular blockade after the paravertebral muscle dissection. A midline incision is made from L1–2 to S1–2, and an L2–L5 osteoplastic laminotomy or laminectomy is performed. The dura is opened and a microscope brought into use. At each level, the anterior (motor) root at each exit foramen is identified, stimulated (usual threshold: 2–3 V, 0.1 s), then protected with a cottonoid strip. The posterior root is divided into 3–8 rootlets, then the sensory threshold is determined for the entire sensory root. That threshold to a 0.1-second stimulus is usually 20–40 V, but may be 80–90 V. The threshold stimulus will elicit a motor response similar in intensity to that induced by stimulation of the motor root with 2–3 V. A train of 50 stimuli for 1 s is then given to the posterior root, and the responses are observed.

Responses considered to be abnormal include (1) clonus; (2) contraction of (ipsilateral) muscles not normally innervated by that nerve; (3) contralateral muscle contraction; (4) clinical or electromyographic contraction that persists after the stimulus ceases, and (5) an electromyographic crescendo pattern during the stimulus. Once the sensory threshold is determined, the individual rootlets are stimulated at the same voltage. Rootlets causing the 'abnormal' responses are divided. If no abnormal responses are seen, the 30–60% of the rootlets causing the strongest tetanic contraction are divided; the decisions about the percentage to divide are based on the intensity of muscle contraction after rootlet stimulation and on the preoperative clinical severity of spasticity in that muscle. The dura is closed, an epidural catheter is inserted for postoperative analgesics, the laminotomy is replaced, and the wound closed.

Postoperative lumbar pain is substantial but is well controlled with epidural morphine (0.05–0.075 mg/kg) every 8–12 h for 2–3 days [12]. Passive range of motion is begun on the 3rd or 4th postoperative day,

Table 1. Definition of Ashworth scores

Ashworth score	Degree of muscle tone
1	No increase in tone
2	Slight increase in tone, giving a 'catch' when affected part is moved in flexion or extension
3	More marked increase in tone; passive movements difficult
4	Considerable increase in tone; passive movements difficult
5	Affected part rigid in flexion or extension

and the patients are discharged 1 week postoperatively. Operative morbidity includes transient bladder dysfunction (5–10%), muscle spasms (<5%), and pain. Operative risks include infection (1%) cerebrospinal fluid leak (2–3%), permanent urinary dysfunction (<1%), hypotonia (<5%), aspiration pneumonia, and bronchospasm (<5%) [9]. The laminotomies and laminectomies required for SPR do not appear to increase the frequency of scoliosis that occurs in children with cerebral palsy.

Relief of spasticity is evident immediately and is thought to be permanent [13]. Physical therapy is needed for months to increase range of motion, to strengthen individual leg muscles, and to improve the gait pattern. The frequency of therapy varies with the postoperative goals. Although the benefits of SPR and its rationale have been recently debated [14], several reports document improved function after SPR.

The muscle tone (Ashworth scale, table 1) in the lower extremities decreases significantly, and the range of motion in the lower extremities is significantly increased [15]. Therapists have demonstrated improved rolling, long-sitting, side-sitting, prone-kneeling, half-kneeling, crawling, standing, and walking [16]. Improved gait, assessed by formal gait analysis, has been documented by Peacock and Staudt [15], Cahan et al. [17], and by our gait laboratory. Improvements include faster gait with a longer stride but with the same cadence, i.e., a more efficient gait. Occupational therapists have demonstrated minor improvements in upper extremity function, an effect perhaps attributable to decreased upper extremity spasticity because of reduced ascending interneuronal inputs.

In summary, SPR is a safe procedure that effectively and probably permanently reduces lower extremity spasticity, improves range of motion, and permits improved function. It is appropriate for patients with spastic diplegia and for those with severe lower extremity spasticity, but is not appropriate for patients who utilize their spasticity to sit, stand, and walk, whose function would deteriorate without it.

Intrathecal Baclofen

The mainstays of medical therapy of spasticity have been baclofen, dantrolene, and diazepam. Medical therapy of spasticity has been ineffective because oral medications cannot be given in adequate quantities to achieve a therapeutic concentration in the spinal cord.

Baclofen, and chlorophenol derivative of the inhibitory neurotransmitter γ-aminobutyric acid (GABA), when given orally is present in the cerebrospinal fluid in concentrations <12 ng/ml [18]. However, the constant intrathecal infusion of 400 μg/day results in cerebrospinal fluid levels of 380 ng/ml, greater than ten times the concentration after oral administration [19]. Intrathecal baclofen infuses into the superficial layers of the spinal cord and binds to $GABA_b$ receptor sites. It acts presynaptically, inhibiting the uptake of calcium and thereby inhibiting the release of excitatory neurotransmitters such as glutamic acid and aspartic acid [20–22].

A single dose of intrathecal baclofen reduces lower extremity muscle tone within 20–40 min. Its maximum effect is seen approximately 4 h after instillation, its half-life is approximately 5 h, and the effects of a single injection are gone within 8–10 h. An overdose of intrathecal baclofen results in coma, respiratory depression, and hypotonia [23], effects that subside over 2–3 days as baclofen is metabolized. Intrathecal baclofen overdoses have been treated with intravenous physostigmine [24] but severe overdoses are not reversed [25].

The use of intrathecal baclofen to treat spasticity of spinal origin was pioneered by Penn and Kroin in 1984 [26]. These authors demonstrated that single intrathecal baclofen doses diminish spinal spasticity in patients with multiple sclerosis. In 1987, Penn and Kroin [23] reported that continuous intrathecal baclofen administered via a programable subcutaneous (Medtronic) pump chronically decreased spasticity in 7 such patients who were unresponsive to oral spasmolytics. In 1989, Penn et al. [27] reported the effects of continuous intrathecal baclofen on lower extremity muscle tone in 20 patients with spinal spasticity secondary to multiple sclerosis or spinal cord injury in a double-blind crossover study. The muscle tone decreased from 4 ± 1.0 to 1.2 ± 0.4, and muscle spasms were decreased in 18 of 19 patients. Continuous intrathecal baclofen maintained normal lower extremity tone for a mean follow-up period of 19.2 months. Penn et al. [27] reported no CNS toxicity, one pump failure, and two catheter-related problems.

The benefits of continuous intrathecal baclofen have been replicated in a European multicenter study and by French and German studies. In the European study, 28 patients with severe spasticity unresponsive to oral medications were treated. Their underlying diseases included multiple sclerosis (n = 12), spinal cord trauma (n = 10), cervical myelopathy (n = 2), and miscellaneous disorders (n = 4). Continuous intrathecal baclofen (50–800 µg/day) completely abolished spasticity with a follow-up of 2 years [28].

In the French study [29] 18 patients were implanted with a Medtronic pump. Sixteen of the patients had spinal spasticity, and 2 had cerebral spasticity. Intrathecal baclofen was given continuously at dosages of 21–500 µg/day (mean 160 µg/day) with a mean follow-up period of 18 months. Spasticity improved in all patients, and muscle spasms resolved in 14 of 16. Functional improvements, measured on a function scale, were observed in 12 of 18 patients. The authors reported 1 overdosage, 3 catheter problems, and 5 patients with either wound sepsis or meningitis. Patients needed only slight increases of baclofen doses during the study.

In the German study [30] (n = 30) patients with spasticity secondary to spinal cord injury (n = 11), multiple sclerosis (n = 11), cerebral palsy (n = 3), or cerebral injury or ischemia (n = 5) were treated with intrathecal baclofen (10–300 µg/day) to determine the efficacy and duration of improvement. They were then implanted with constant-infusion (Infusaid) pumps and treated with 10–900 µg (mean 333 µg/day). The mean follow-up period was 10 months. The Ashworth scores in the lower extremities decreased from 4.3 ± 0.8 (before treatment) to 1.5 ± 0.69 (after treatment), painful spasms were eliminated in 13 of 17 patients, and the integrated electromyogram decreased by 55%. Catheter, wound, or injection port complications required minor surgery in 8 patients, and meningitis occured in 2.

The effects of intrathecal baclofen on voluntary motor control in 6 patients with spinal spasticity were reported by Latash et al. [31]. These authors measured the electromyographic activity in agonist and antagonist lower extremity muscles and found that, prior to baclofen injections, agonists and antagonists fired simultaneously. After single baclofen doses (50–75 μg), the antagonist interference was markedly suppressed.

The effects of intrathecal baclofen injections in children with cerebral palsy were recently reported [32]. In that randomized, double-blind study, 17 patients with congenital spastic cerebral palsy and 6 patients with other forms of hypertonicity, who were not candidates for SPR, were injected intrathecally with single baclofen doses (25–100 μg). Many of the patients used some spasticity to stand and walk. Muscle tone in the upper and lower extremities was graded on the Ashworth scale by physical therapists before each injection and 2 h afterward for 8 h; the upper-extremity function was assessed by occupational therapists before and 4 h after each injection. The muscle tone in the lower extremities decreased significantly within 4 h after all intrathecal baclofen doses and remained reduced for 8 h; upper extremity tone and function were not affected by the single doses.

Programmable subcutaneous (Medtronic) pumps have been implanted into 19 children with cerebral palsy whose mean lower extremity spasticity was decreased by 1.0 or more (Ashworth scale) after single intrathecal baclofen injections. Continuous intrathecal baclofen (25–400 μg/day) has been infused for 1 year or longer in 9 and the decrease in muscle tone seen after single injections has been maintained by continuous infusions. Many of these patients need some spasticity to stand, to transfer, or to walk; the goal of therapy has been to titrate the intrathecal baclofen dosage so that spasticity is diminished but not abolished. The lower extremity muscle tone (Ashworth scale) has decreased 1.0 or greater in 8/9. Occupational therapists have documented improved activities of daily living in 7 of 9 and improved grasps in 3 of 9 patients. Decreased upper extremity muscle tone and increased range of motion have been seen routinely in patients treated with continuous intrathecal baclofen.

Continuous intrathecal baclofen is best accomplished via a pump, the infusion rate of which can be externally adjusted. The initial continuous infusion dose is usually twice the single intrathecal dose that produces a clinically significant response (i.e., $\leq$1.0 decrease in average lower extremity tone). The daily dose is adjusted slowly upward over the first 2–3 months until the desired effects are present. Pumps are refilled by percutaneous injections every 3 months. Dosages have varied little after the first 3 months in patients with cerebral palsy followed up to 2.5 years.

Rhizotomy or Baclofen

Although both SPR and intrathecal baclofen effectively treat spasticity, they each have advantages and disadvantages and appear to have different indications. Children on the mild end of the spastic cerebral palsy spectrum are probably best treated by SPR; their therapy can be definitive. Children in the middle of the spectrum, with spastic quadriparesis, who use their spasticity to stand and walk, are best treated by intrathecal baclofen because its effects can be titrated. Children on the severe end of the spasticity spectrum can be treated with either SPR or intrathecal baclofen; SPR lower extremity benefits will be permanent but intrathecal baclofen will improve both upper and lower extremity tone. Patients with unilateral spasticity are probabliy not candidates for intrathecal baclofen which would presumably diminish muscle tone on the normal side as well as on the side with spasticity.

References

1 Sherrington CS: Decerebrate rigidity and reflex coordination of movements. J Physiol (Lond) 1898;22:319–337.
2 Foerster O: On the indications and results of the excision of posterior spinal nerve roots in men. Surg Gynecol Obstet 1913;5:463–474.
3 Gros C, Frèrebeau PH, Kuhner A, Perez-Dominguez E: Technical modification in the Foerster operation. Selective posterior lumbar root section. The results of 18 years of practice. 5th int Congr of Neurosurgery, Tokyo 1973.
4 Sindou M, Fischer G, Mansuy L: Posterior spinal rhizotomy and selective posterior rhizidiotomy. Prog Neurol Surg 1976;7:201–250.
5 Fasano VA: Surgical treatment of spasticity in cerebral palsy. Childs Brain 1978; 4:289–305.
6 Laitenen LV, Nilsson S, Fugl-Meyer AR: Selective posterior rhizotomy for treatment of spasticity. J Neurosurg 1989;58:895–899.
7 Peacock WJ, Arens LJ, Berman B: Cerebral palsy spasticity: Selective posterior rhizotomy. Pediatr Neurosci 1987;13:61–66.
8 Cahan LD, Kundi SM, McPherson D: Electrophysiologic studies in selective posterior rhizotomy for spasticity in children with cerebral palsy. Appl Neurophysiol 1987;50:459–460.

9 Abbott R, Forem SL, Johann M: Selective posterior rhizotomy for the treatment of spasticity: A review. Childs Nerv Syst 1989;5:337–346.

10 Albright AL: Selective posterior rhizotomies for spasticity in children. J Prosthet Orthot 1989:2:54–58.

11 Lazareff JA, Mata-Acosta AM, Garcia-Mendez MA: Limited selective posterior rhizotomy for the treatment of spasticity secondary to infantile cerebral palsy: A preliminary report. Neurosurgery 1990;27:535–538.

12 Sparks ML, Klein AL, Duhaime AC, Mickle JP: Use of epidural morphine for control of postoperative pain in selective dorsal rhizotomy for spasticity. Pediatr Neurosci 1989;15:229–232.

13 Arens LJ, Peacock WJ, Peter J: Selective posterior rhizotomy: A long-term follow-up study. Childs Nerv Syst 1989;5:148–152.

14 Landau WM, Hunt CC: Dorsal rhizotomy, a treatment of unproved efficacy. J Child Neurol 1990;5:174–178.

15 Peacock WJ, Staudt LA: Functional outcomes following selective posterior rhizotomy in children with cerebral palsy. J Neurosurg 1991;74:380–375.

16 Berman B, Vaughan CL, Peacock WJ: The effect of rhizotomy on movement in patients with cerebral palsy. Am J Occup Ther 1989;44:511–516.

17 Cahan LD, Beeler L, Adams J, et al: Gait analysis after selective posterior rhizotomy (abstract). Pediatric Selection, American Association of Neurological Surgery, Scottsdale, December 1988.

18 Knutsson E, Lindblom U, Martensson A: Plasma and cerebrospinal fluid levels of baclofen (Lioresal) at optimal therapeutic responses in spastic paresis. J Neurol Sci 1974;23:473–484.

19 Müller H, Zierski J, Dralle D, Kraus D, Mutschuler E: Pharmacokinetics of intrathecal baclofen; in Müller H, Zierski J, Penn RD (eds): Local-Spinal Therapy of Spasticity. New York, Springer, 1988, pp 223–226.

20 Zeiglgansberger W, Howe JR, Sutor B: The neuropharmacology of baclofen; in Müller H, Zierski J, Penn RD (eds): Local-Spinal Therapy of Spasticity. New York, Springer, 1988, pp 37–49.

21 Delwaide PJ, Young RR: Drug therapy. Spasticity 1981;304:28–33, 96–99.

22 Bowery NG, Hill DR, Hudson AL, et al: Baclofen decreases neurotransmitter release in the mammalian CNS by an action at a novel GABA receptor. Nature 1980;283:92–94.

23 Penn RD, Kroin JS: Long-term intrathecal baclofen for treatment of spasticity. J Neurosurg 1987;66:181–185.

24 Müller-Schwefe G, Penn RD: Physostigmine in the treatment of intrathecal baclofen overdose: Report of three cases. J Neurosurg 1989;71:273–275.

25 Saltuaria L, Baumgartner H, Kefler M, et al: Failure of physostigmine in treatment of acute severe intrathecal baclofen intoxication. N Engl J Med 1990; 322:1535.

26 Penn RD, Kroin JS: Intrathecal baclofen alleviates spinal cord spasticity. Lancet 1984;i:1078.

27 Penn RD, Savoy SM, Corcos D, et al: Intrathecal baclofen for severe spinal spasticity. N Engl J Med 1989;320:1517–1521.

28 Gochs, Struppler A, Meyerson BA, Linderoth B, Gybels J, Gardner BP, Teddy P, Jamous A, Weinman P: Intrathecal baclofen for long-term treatment of

spasticity: A multi-centre study. J Neurol Neurosurg Psychiatry 1989;52: 933–939.
29 Lazothes Y, Sallerin-Daute B, Verdie JC, Bastide R, Carillo JP: Chronic intrathecal baclofen administration for control of severe spasticity. J Neurosurg 1990;72: 393–403.
30 Zierski J, Müller H, Dralle D, et al: Implanted pump systems for treatment of spasticity. Acta Neurochir (Wien) 1988;43(suppl):94–99.
31 Latash ML, Penn RD, Corcos DM, Gottlieb GL: Effects of intrathecal baclofen on voluntary motor control in spastic paresis. J Neurosurg 1990;72:388–392.
32 Albright AL, Cervi A, Singletary J: Intrathecal baclofen for spasticity in cerebral palsy. JAMA 1991;265:1418–1422.

A. Leland Albright, MD, Department of Neurosurgery, Children's Hospital, University of Pittsburgh School of Medicine, Pittsburgh, Pa. (USA)

Proceedings of the Meeting of the American Society for Stereotactic and Functional Neurosurgery, Pittsburgh, Pa., June 16–19, 1991
Stereotact Funct Neurosurg 1992;58:14–21

Ventroposterolateral Pallidotomy Can Abolish All Parkinsonian Symptoms

L.V. Laitinen, A.T. Bergenheim, M.I. Hariz

Departement of Neurosurgery, Sophiahemmet Hospital, Stockholm, and University Hospital, Umeå, Sweden

Key Words. Parkinson's disease · Tremor · Rigidity · Hyporkinesia · Stereotactic surgery · Pallidotomy

Abstract. Stereotactic ventroposterolateral pallidotomy in 46 parkinsonian patients resulted in a complete or almost complete and long-lasting relief of rigidity and hypokinesia in 91% of the patients. Good tremor effect was obtained in 80% of them. The *L*-dopa-induced dyskinesias, gait and speech improved in most patients. Complications were observed in 7 cases after 51 pallidotomies, i.e. 14% (partial homonymous hemianopia in 6 and transient dysphasia and facial weakness in 1). We belive that the good effect of surgery is based on interruption of some striopallidal or subthalamopallidal pathways.

In 1960 Svennilson et al. [1] reported that stereotactic lesions in the ventroposterolateral (VPL) pallidum had abolished all three cardinal symptoms of Parkinson's disease, i.e., tremor, rigidity and bradykinesia, and that the effect had been long-lasting. In the late 1950s, the neurosurgeons had already begun to operate in the ventrolateral (VL) thalamus, and the revolutionary pallidotomy developed by Lars Leksell in 1956–1957 fell into oblivion. Thalamotomy in the VL and ventral intermediate (Vim) nuclei proved to be effective against parkinsonian tremor, but it made the bradykinesia worse [2]. Most neurologists were aware of this, and seldom referred parkinsonian patients for surgery.

During the last decade increasing neurophysiological evidence indicated that the parkinsonian symptoms, inclusive of akinesia, might be due to striopallidal or striosubthalamopallidal hyperactivity [3–5]. There was reason to pesume that Leksell's successful VPL pallidotomy had interrupted such pathways. In 1985 we began to use this approach

1011–6125/92/0584–0014 $ 2.75/0

Table 1. VPL pallidotomy 1985–April 1991

Target	Patients n	Operations n
Right pallidum	17	17
Left pallidum	12	12
Bilateral pallidum	5	10
Right pallidum and left thalamus	8	16
Left pallidum and right thalamus	2	4
Left pallidum and bilateral thalamus	2	6
Total	46	65

in parkinsonian patients who were not considered to be candidates for thalamotomy. A preliminary study on 38 patients showed that all parkinsonian symptoms could be abolished by VPL pallidotomy [6]. In this paper we present a larger patient material and discuss the possible mechanisms of surgery.

Patients and Methods

From 1985 to April 1991, VPL pallidotomy was carried out in 46 parkinsonian patients who suffered from severe tremor, rigor, bradykinesia, gait difficulties and/or dyskinesias with muscle pain. Pure bradykinesia, without or with little tremor, was often the dominating symptom. The age of the patients ranged from 30 to 80 (mean 60.1) years. The duration of illness ranged from 2 to 20 (mean 9.3) years. All patients had received physiotherapy and conventional drug therapy, but the effect had not been satisfactory.

Pallidotomy was unilateral in 41 and bilateral in 5 patients. Ten patients had previously had thalamotomy on one side and pallidotomy was done on the other side. Two patients had previously had bilateral thalamotomies. Thus, the total number of operations was 65 (table 1).

The pallidal target was defined by stereotactic CT with Laitinen's stereoadapter [7]. The target coordinates were: 2–3 mm in front of the midcommissural point; 6 mm below the intercommissural line (the ventralmost position of the electrode tip), and 18–22 mm lateral to the midline of the third ventricle. Laitinen's stereotactic system [7] was used. Through a frontal burr hole lying 2 cm lateral to the sagittal suture, a 1.8-mm-thick monopolar electrode with a 2-mm-long uninsulated tip was introduced under local anesthesia to the target. The final lesion site was based on impedance recording and electrical stimulation.

Table 2. Threshold responses to electrical stimulation of VPL pallidum (60 Hz, 2–5 mA): clinical side effects

Response	Cases n	Side effect
Increased muscle tension	17	
Visual phenomenon	13	homonymous scotoma 6
Tremor increase	14	
Tremor decrease	5	
Nausea	5	
Paresthesiae	4	
Muscular jerks	2	hemiparesis 2
Speech arrest	2	dysphasia 1
Anxiety	1	
None	4	

Electrical stimulation parameteres were: rectangular monophasic 1-ms-long pulses, 60 and 6 Hz, intensity 2–10 mA. The threshold responses to pallidal stimulation generally required higher current intensity than those to VL-VIM thalamic stimulation. Threshold reponses to 60 Hz stimulation are shown in table 2.

Radiofrequency thermolesions were so planned that the dorsoventral length of the lesion presumably would be 6–7 mm and the transverse diameter about 6 mm. When electrical stimulation gave visual responses, the final lesion was often made more dorsally than originally planned and its size was reduced.

The akinesia was assessed with the Purdue pegboard test, a writing, drawing and gait test, 1 day before and 1 day after surgery.

Results

All patients tolerated the surgery well. They were mobilized immediately after surgery and could have a meal. They left the hospital on the following day. At the follow-up examination 2–78 months (mean 30 months) later, a complete or almost complete tremor relief was observed in 80% of them; 91% had a good relief of rigidity and hypokinesia (table 3). The gait and the speech volume, as well as the *L*-dopa-induced involuntary movements and muscular pain also showed remarkable improvement (table 4). The drugs were often gradually reduced to about 50% of the preoperative level. Two patients with severe anxiety of long duration experienced a good emotional improvement.

Table 3. Effect of VPL pallidotomy on tremor, rigidity and hypokinesia in 46 patients

Degree	Tremor		Rigor		Hypokinesia	
	pre	post	pre	post	pre	post
Nil	11	28	–	22	–	23
Slight	7	12	3	20	1	19
Moderate	17	5	29	4	22	3
Severe	11	1	14	–	23	1

pre = Before operation; post = after operation.

Table 4. Effect of VPL pallidotomy on gait, speech and dystonia/pain in 46 patients

Degree of Dysfunction	Gait		Speech		Dystonia/pain	
	pre	post	pre	post	pre	post
Nil	1	13	22	28	15	31
Slight	8	25	13	13	10	11
Moderate	23	7	8	5	10	4
Severe	14	1	3	–	11	–

pre = Before operation; post = after operation.

Postoperative stereotactic CT was done 3–12 months later in 15 patients to check the size and the site of the lesions. They laid in the posteroventrolateral region of the pallidum, very close to the amygdala and the internal capsule. Their size ranged from 21 to 180 mm^3, with a mean of 98 mm^3.

Complications were observed in 7 patients after 51 pallidotomies. Six (12%) had a central lower quadrant homonymous scotoma. One of them also had a transient dysphasia and facial weakness. One patient had a minor vascular accident with transitory hemiparesis 1 week after surgery, but later made a good recovery.

Discussion

Our study confirmed the findings of Svennilson et al. [1] that parkinsonian tremor, rigor and hypokinesia can be effectively abolished by VPL pallidotomy. Also the *L*-dopa-induced involuntary movements and painful muscle cramps react well. The effect seems to be long-lasting. The general effect of VPL pallidotomy is clearly better than that obtained with VL/VIM thalamotomy. Thalamotomy is well known to abolish the parkinsonian tremor. Its effect on the rigidity is also good, whereas the bradykinesia usually becomes worse [2]. It is also well known that the gait seldom improves. The thalamotomized patient often tilts toward the side contralateral to surgery and this side lags behind the more healthy side. The balance, the speech volume and the articulation often suffer from unilateral thalamotomy. These side effects are almost constant after bilateral thalamotomy.

The classical pallidotomy with lesions in the anterodorsal and medial part of the pallidum, as reported in 1958 by Cooper and Bravo [8] only seems to have improved the rigidity, but very little the tremor. Little was written about its effect on the bradykinesia.

There is increasing experimental and clinical evidence indicating that all parkinsonian symptoms, at least the tremor and bradykinesia, and presumably also the rigidity develop in, or are mediated by, the pallidum or subthalamopallidal region [1–5]. Dopamine deficiency in the putamen presumably leads to an inhibitory GABAergic hyperactivity in the direct striopallidal pathway, which in the anterior and dorsomedial part of the pallidum blocks the initiation of movement and causes akinesia. Tremor and rigidity also are related to dopamine deficiency and an imbalance in striosubthalamopallidal pathways [5]. We hypothesize that the medial pallidum may function as a traffic control station which via the pallidothalamocortical ascending pathways gives the cortical motor cells a green light signal for initiation and execution of movements. Pallidal inhibition switches on a red light signal and freezing of the voluntary movements, i.e. akinesia occurs. Rhythmic inhibition may lead to rigidity and resting tremor (fig. 1). Dopamine hyperactivity in the striatum leads to a decreased inhibition on the medial pallidum, with choreic/hemiballistic movements as a result.

Surgical lesions in the striopallidal output pathways, i.e., the medial pallidum, ansa and fasciculus lenticularis, or in the VL thala-

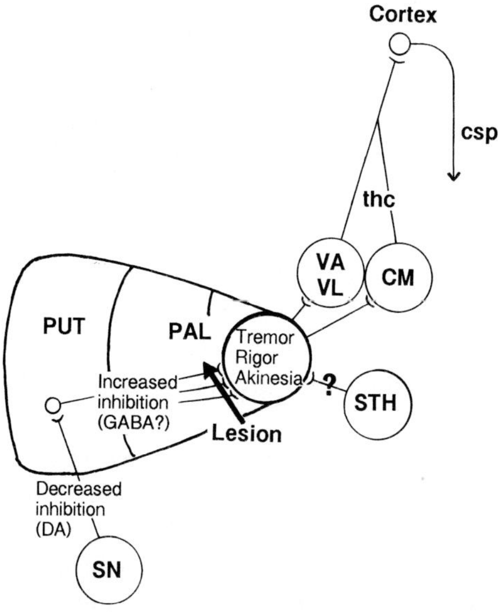

Fig. 1. Presumed action mechanism of VPL pallidotomy on parkinsonian symptoms. The lesion in the part VPL of the pallidum (PAL) interrupts the direct GABAergic striopallidal pathway which due to striatal dopamine (DA) deficiency exerts an increased inhibitory effect on the medial pallidum, where all parkinsonian symptoms (tremor, rigor, akinesia) are supposed to develop as release phenomena. The disturbances are mediated along the striopallidal main output pathways via the ventral anterior (VA) and VL nuclei of the thalamus to the premotor and motor cortex. The subthalamic nucleus (STH) may through indirect striosubthalamopallidal mechanisms play a role in the development of the symptoms [5]. SN = Substantia nigra; PUT = putameri; CM = Centrum medianum; thc = Thalamocortical; csp = Corticospinal.

mus can therefore only block the tremor and rigidity, but at the same time they worsen the initiation of movement [2].

Recently, we have in several parkinsonian patients observed small localized calcifications in the anterodorsal medial pallidum [unpubl. data] which is further evidence that this portion of the pallidum is pathological in Parkinson's disease.

As was shown by Svennilson et al. [1] and ourselves [6], stereotactic lesions in the lateral part of the posteroventral pallidum can abolish all parkinsonian symptoms. The *L*-dopa-induced involuntary movements also disappear. Lesions in the same target also alleviate hemiballism [9]. Similar effects have recently been documented in MPTP-treated animals with lesions in the subthalamic nucleus [5]. Therefore, it seems likely that our lesions in the VPL pallidum interrupt some striopallidal or striosubthalamopallidal pathways and re-establish more or less normal motor functioning in parkinsonian patients.

All this proves that the parkinsonian akinesia is a reversible condition. Babinski et al. demonstrated in 1921 [10] that severely akinetic parkinsonian patients were able to start a nearly normal performance when confronted with strong emotional stimuli. They called the phenomenon 'kinésie paradoxale'. *L*-Dopa therapy has also proved that akinesia is reversible.

The only serious side effect of VPL pallidotomy consists of a hemianoptic defect in the lower central visual field contralateral to surgery. The defect is presumably due to a heat lesion of the dorsolateral aspect of the optic tract. The defect is perceived by the patients as a small shadow or spot. It is easily observed by the patient, and in a perimetry study, but it cannot be detected in a clinical visual confrontation test. In 5 patients the field defect on the left side did not disturb very much, but in the 6th patient the small central defect on the right side was very troublesome, because it made reading difficult. The defect seems to be permanent.

In all 6 patients who had the hemianoptic complication, the effect of surgery on the parkinsonian symptoms was excellent. This indicates that the optimal pallidal target has to be located in the most ventral part of the pallidum, lateral to the optic tract.

In those patients where the clinical effect of surgery was not good, the lesion was small and located in a more dorsal region of the posterior pallidum. Such a placement of the lesion was due to inexperience in the early stage of our practice of pallidotomy, or to an optic tract response to electrical stimulation. In the latter case we withdrew the probe in a dorsal direction, until stimulation no more gave visual responses. At the present time, if an optic response occurs, we reposition the probe in a lateral direction, but keep the ventral level unchanged.

The shape of the lesion may ultimately play an important role. Leksell's very large lesions were disk-shaped, flat in anteroposterior directions, whereas our lesions were much smaller and spherical. If the beneficial effect of the lesions is based on interruption of a pathway, as we believe, it would be logical to test which shape is most effective.

Conclusions

(1) In most parkinsonian patients, VPL pallidotomy abolishes all symptoms contralateral to surgery. The effect is long-lasting. (2) Unilateral severe drug-resistant bradykinesia with dystonia and muscular pain, particularly in the legs, is the best indication for surgery. The tremor, rigidity and the *L*-dopa-induced choreoathetosis also react well to pallidotomy. The drug therapy can often be reduced after surgery. (3) The lesions must be placed in a close vicinity to the optic tract, which implies a great risk for central homonymous hemianopia. Other side-effects are rare. (4) We believe that the good effect of VPL pallidotomy is based on interruption of some striopallidal or striosubthalamopallidal pathways.

References

1 Svennilson E, Torvik A, Lowe R, Leksell L: Treatment of Parkinsonism by stereotactic thermolesions in the pallidal region. Acta Psychiatr Neurol Scand 1960;35:358–377.
2 Laitinen L, Vilkki J: Measurement of parkinsonian hypokinesia with Purdue pegboard and motor reaction time tests; in Siegfried J (ed): Parkinson's Disease. Berlin, Huber, 1973, vol 2, pp 185–192.
3 Iansek R: The effects of reserpine on motor activity and pallidal discharge in monkeys: Implications for the genesis of akinesia. J Physiol 1980;301:457–466.
4 Iansek R, Porter R: The monkey globus pallidus: Neuronal discharge properties in relation to movement. J Physiol 1980;301:439–455.
5 DeLong MR: Primate models of movement disorders of basal ganglia origin. Trends Neurosci 1990;13:281–285.
6 Laitinen LV, Bergenheim AT, Hariz MI: Leksell's posteroventral pallidotomy in the treatment of Parkinson's disease. J Neurosurg, in press.
7 Laitinen LV: Noninvasive multipurpose stereoadapter. Neurol Res 1987;9:137–141.
8 Cooper IS, Bravo G: Chemopallidectomy and chemothalamectomy. J Neurosurg 1958;15:244–250.
9 Tsubokawa T, Moriyasu N: Lateral pallidotomy for relief of ballistic movement: Its basic evidences and clinical application. Confin Neurol 1975;37:10–15.
10 Babinski J, Jarkowski B, Plichet V: Kinésie paradoxale. Mutisme parkinsonien. Rev Neurol 1921;37:1266–1270.

Lauri V. Laitinen, MD, PhD, Sophiahemmet Hospital, PO Box 5605,
S–11486 Stockholm (Sweden)

Proceedings of the Meeting of the American Society for Stereotactic and Functional Neurosurgery, Pittsburgh, Pa., June 16–19, 1991
Stereotact Funct Neurosurg 1992;58:22–25

Stereotactic Thalamotomy for Medically Intractable Essential Tremor

Marc S. Goldman, Patrick J. Kelly

Department of Neurosurgery, Mayo Clinic, Rochester, Minn., USA

Key Words. Stereotaxis · Thalamotomy · Essential tremor · Functional outcome · Movement disorder · Voice tremor

Abstract. Objective surgical symptomatic outcome of ventrolateral (VL) thalamotomy specifically for essential tremor is uncommonly reported and functional outcome has not been investigated previously. In the present series, 7 patients underwent unilateral and 1 patient staged bilateral VL thalamotomies for disabling medically refractory essential tremor. At follow-up examination (mean 17.3 months, range 1–50 months), all patients enjoyed complete ablation or significant amelioration of the targeted tremor. Disability as determined by a modified form of an established rating scale for tremor was reduced from moderate (57%) or severe (43%) to absent (86%) or mild (14%). Interestingly, voice tremor was ablated or significantly improved in 71.4% of patients with preoperative voice tremor.

Objective surgical symptomatic outcome of ventrolateral (VL) thalamotomy specifically for essential tremor is uncommonly reported and functional outcome has not been investigated previously. This series explored the symptomatic and functional impact of VL thalamotomy on patients with unequivocal disabling essential tremor.

Patients and Methods

Patients

At the Mayo Clinic, from September 1984 to March 1991, 9 stereotactic thalamotomies were performed on 8 patients for disabling unequivocal essential tremor. One patient received staged bilateral stereotactic thalamotomies for bilateral severe tremor.

1011–6125/92/0584–0022 $ 2.75/0

General neurological examinations, psychometric evaluations, speech pathology evaluations and neuroradiologic scans (CT and/or MRI) were performed preoperatively, and repeated during the first postoperative week, at the patient's first postoperative follow-up appointment (3 months) and at successive visits as circumstances permitted. Videotaped documentation of the tremor and selected segments of the neurological examination were performed preoperatively and at each postsurgical evaluation. Tremor was graded on a 4-point scale (0 = none; 4 = severe) with respect to each component: rest, static, action and terminal accentuation.

The mean age of the 8 patients was 46.4 years (range 18–69 years) at the time of operation. All of the patients were male. Positive family histories of tremor were present in all cases where obtainable (1 patient was adopted). Stereotactic VL thalamotomies were performed on the left in 6 (75%) patients, on the right in 1 (12.5%) patient, and 1 patient (12.5%) received staged bilateral thalamotomies at a 6-month interval. Preoperative and postoperative disability was graded in 7 patients according to a modified form of the clinical rating scale for tremor by Fahn et al. [1]. One patient was unavailable for disability determination.

The disability scale represented the composite score of a 4-point grading system (0 = normal; 4 = severe disability) which evaluated specific areas of function: handwriting, speaking, solid and liquid feeding, hygiene, dressing and employment.

Postoperative neurological morbidity was defined as a new deficit or worsened preoperative deficit and was labeled transient or persistent depending on its presence at the most recent follow-up examination.

Surgical Procedure

Utilizing the COMPASS™ stereotactic system (Stereotactic Medical Systems, New Hartford, N.Y., USA), the VL thalamus was targeted. The coordinates of the junction of the ventral intermediate/(Vim)/ventro-oralis posterior VOP thalamus corresponding to the receptive fields in the ventroposterior thalamus of the contralateral buccal commissure and thumb were estimated utilizing a computer resident Schaltenbrand-Wahren stereotactic atlas superimposed on stereotactic CT and MRI scans and Guiot-Talairach constructs based on anteroposterior and lateral stereotactic ventriculograms. The target was then precisely localized with microelectrode recording and stimulation control. Radiofrequency lesions were made with a 1.6-mm probe as desribed in detail elsewhere [2, 3].

Results

Tremor

There was complete immediate ablation of the contralateral targeted upper extremity tremor in all 9 thalamotomies. Follow-up examination (mean 17.3 months, range 1–50 months) disclosed complete ablation (4 patients) or significant amelioration (3 patients) in all patients undergoing unilateral thalamotomy. The patient undergoing

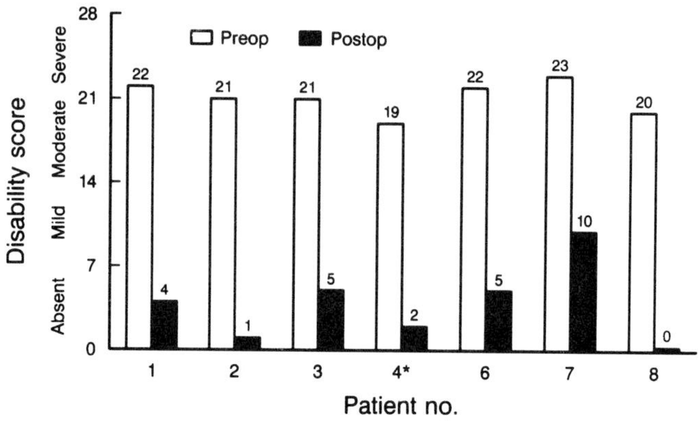

Fig. 1. Preoperative and postoperative disability scores after VL thalamotomy for medically intractable disabling essential tremor. Patient No. 4: final score after second of staged bilateral thalamotomies.

staged bilateral thalamotomies experienced complete abolition of his dominant tremor and near-complete abolition of his nondominant tremor. At a mean follow-up interval of 19 months (range 1–50 months), disability was reduced from a mean score of 21.1 to a mean score of 3.9 ($p < 0.001$; fig. 1).

Speech

Seven of the 8 patients demonstrated voice tremor preoperatively. At follow-up, 5 patients (71.4%) experienced ablation (3 patients) or improvement (2 patients) in voice tremor.

Morbidity

There was no operative mortality and no severe persistent operative morbidity. A mild persistent dysarthria was found in 2 patients, and mild persistent verbal cognitive deficit was found in 1 patient. All patients experiencing persistent deficits were either older than 65 (2 patients) or underwent staged bilateral procedures (1 patient). There was no clear correlation between side of lesion and persistent postoperative deficit.

Conclusions

In this series, 8 cases of unequivocal essential tremor underwent VL thalamotomy. There was complete or near-complete ablation of tremor in all patients. There was no surgical mortality, and persistent neurological morbidity was uncommon and mild. Disability was reduced from a mean score of 21 (moderate grade) to a mean score of 3.9 (absent grade). Stereotactic VL thalamotomy for medically intractable debilitating essential tremor carries a low surgical risk and is a dramatically effective treatment option for this group of patients.

References

1 Fahn S, Tolosa E, Martin C: Clinical rating scale for tremor; in Jankovic J, Tolosa E (eds): Parkinson's Disease and Movement Disorders. Baltimore, Urban & Schwarzenberg, 1988, pp 225–234.
2 Kelly PJ: Principles of stereotactic surgery: Instrumentation and procedural aspects; in Youmans JR (ed): Neurological Surgery, ed 3. Philadelphia, Saunders, 1990, vol 6, pp 4183–4226.
3 Kelly PJ, Ahlskog JE, Goerss SJ, Daube JR, Duffy JR, Kall BA: Computer assisted stereotactic ventralis thalamotomy with microelectrode recording control in patients with Parkinson's disease. Mayo Clin Proc 1987;62:655–664.

Patrick J. Kelly, MD, Department of Neurosurgery, Mayo Clinic, Rochester, MN 55905 (USA)

Proceedings of the Meeting of the American Society for Stereotactic and Functional Neurosurgery, Pittsburgh, Pa., June 16–19, 1991
Stereotact Funct Neurosurg 1992;58:26–29

Ventral Intermediate Thalamotomy for Posttraumatic Hemiballismus

M.F. Lévesque, Charles H. Markham

Division of Neurosurgery and Department of Neurology, UCLA School of Medicine, Los Angeles, Calif., USA

Key Words. Hemiballismus · Head injury · Stereotactic thalamotomy · Subthalamic nucleus

Abstract. An unusual case of hemiballismus following closed head injury is presented. The abnormal movement persisted for 16 years despite medical treatment. Preoperative studies did not reveal a specific lesion within the subthalamic nucleus or within the basal ganglia. A stereotactic ventral intermediate thalamotomy was performed producing a complete resolution of the ballistic movement which persisted for the length of our 12-month follow-up.

Introduction

Hemiballismus is one of the most unusual dyskinesias. It is characterized as unilateral involuntary movement of the proximal extremities and is usually associated with a lesion within the contralateral subthalamic nucleus (STN). Posttraumatic hemiballismus is one of the rarest causes of hemiballismus. We report a case that was treated effectively by stereotactic ventral intermediate thalamotomy.

Case Report

This 39-year-old left-handed male sustained a serious closed head injury at age 15. This was followed by a prolonged coma for 3 weeks. While coming out of the comatose state he began to develop a constant left upper extremity flinging movement involving the proximal musculature of the arm and shoulder. This was abolished during sleep and was not modified by alcohol ingestion. There was no related torticollis or blepharospasm, and his family history was negative for dystonia. Neurological examination

1011–6125/92/0584–0026 $ 2.75/0

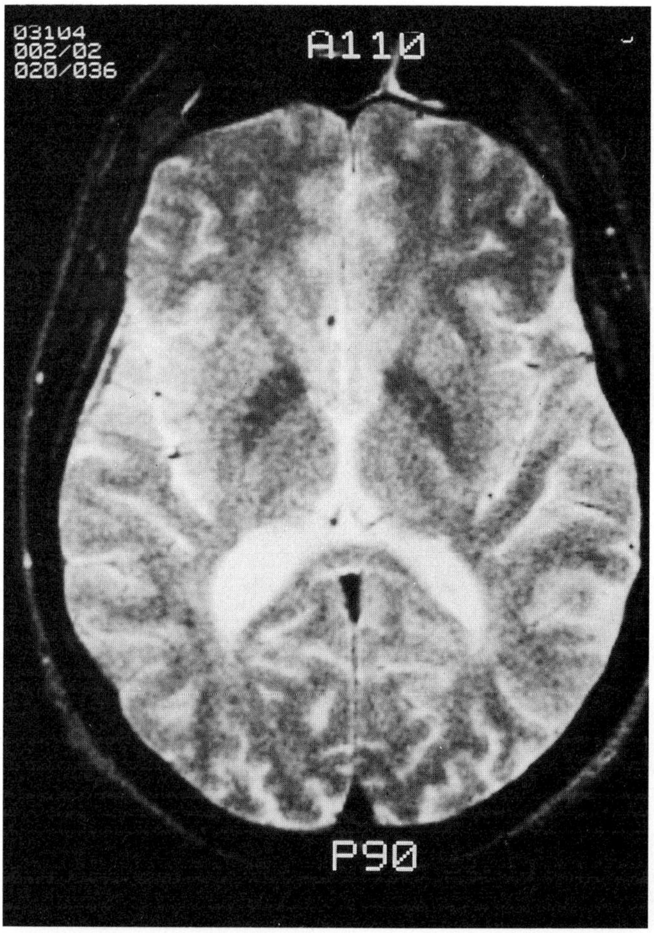

Fig. 1. Preoperative axial T2-weighted MRI of the patient with posttraumatic hemiballismus. Basal ganglion and subthalamus have a normal appearance.

demonstrated a persistent involuntary movement of the left upper extremity involving the proximal more than the distal muscles with the arm flinging up and down in an erratic fashion. There was no fasciculation or weakness. The neck and head were intermittently involved and there was no palatal myoclonus. Mental status was normal with no cognitive deficit. Neurological examination showed increased tone in the right upper extremity and a mild hypotonia with normal strength in the left upper extremity. Both lower extremities were normal. Neurological imaging studies with CT and MRI

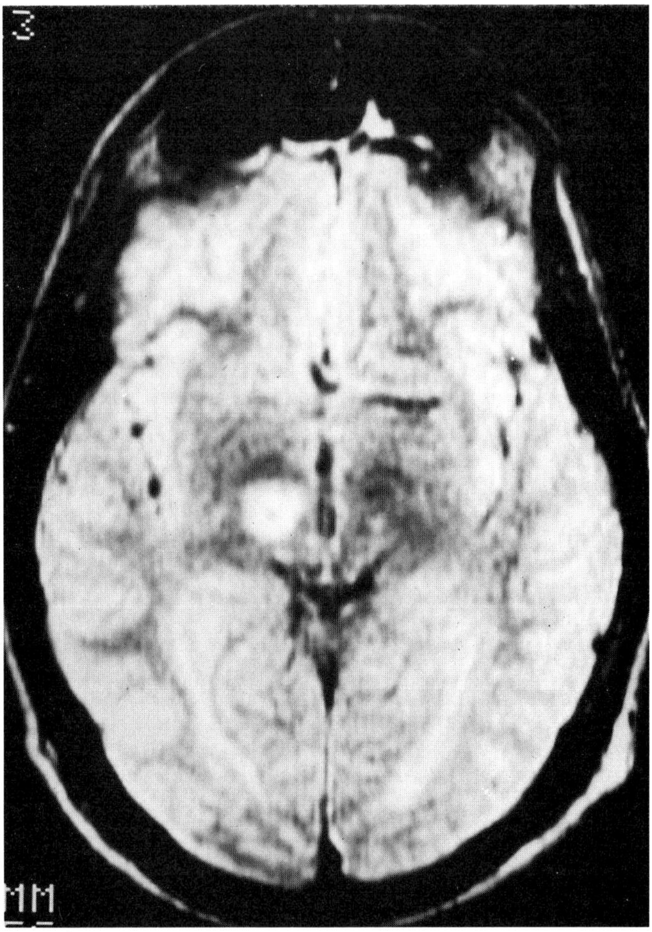

Fig. 2. Postoperative MRI of the same patient 5 days following ventral intermediate thalamotomy. The perilesional edema indicates the satisfactory localization within the VL thalamus in relation to the third ventricle.

were normal (fig. 1). The patient underwent a right-sided ventrolateral (VL) thalamotomy under local anesthesia. After neurophysiological localization, a 70 °C lesion was created for 90 s. There was no postoperative complication. There was a significant improvement in the ballistic movements which completely resolved 2 weeks following surgery. The patient developed mild cerebellar ataxia in the left upper extremity and some slurring of speech. Postoperative MRI showed a well-circumscribed lesion measuring 1 cm in diameter within the right VL thalamus (fig. 2).

Discussion

Hemiballismus usually presents with a violent flinging movement of the extremities associated with mild hypotonia. It is usually associated with a vascular lesion in the subthalamic nucleus as described [1]. Experimental hemiballismus has been produced in animals by stereotactic lesion of the STN. It is now believed that the main efferents from the STN to the globus pallidus are excitatory (glutamatergic). Thus, this pathway modulates the efferent inhibitory output from the globus pallidus to the thalamus. A lesion within the STN would result in a disinhibition of thalamocortical projections and explain the dyskinesia. Recent reports have described lesions outside the STN, involving the neostriatum, that could also produce a combination of hemiballismus or hemichorea [2].

Previous surgical treatments varied from surgical ablation of the brachial plexus, amputation of the affected limb or resection of cerebral motor cortex. Stereotactic VL thalamotomy was felt to produce the best results until new pharmacological agents were introduced [3]. Medical therapy now is aimed at modulating dopamine activity with phenothiazines or reserpine. Recently, some improvement of the hemiballismus with GABAergic agents has been described [4]. Our case is unique because the patient did not respond to medical therapy and he did not have an obvious lesion on neuroimaging studies. Stereotactic lesioning produced excellent results and is indicated when medical therapy fails.

References

1 Jakob A: Die extrapyramidalen Erkrankungen. Berlin, Springer, 1923, pp 183–225.
2 Lownie SP, Gilbert JJ: Hemichorea and hemiballismus: Recent concepts. Clin Neuropathol 1990;9:46–50.
3 Martin JP, McCaul IR: Acute hemiballismus treated by ventrolateral thalamolysis. Brain 1959;82:104–108.
4 Shannon KM: Hemiballismus. Clin Neuropharmacol 1990;13:413–425.

M.F. Lévesque, Division of Neurosurgery, UCLA School of Medicine, 760 Westwood Plaza, Los Angeles, CA 90024 (USA)

Proceedings of the Meeting of the American Society for Stereotactic and Functional Neurosurgery, Pittsburgh, Pa., June 16–19, 1991
Stereotact Funct Neurosurg 1992;58:30–32

Magnetic Resonance Imaging and Anatomic Atlas Mapping for Thalamotomy

T.L. Hardy, J.R. Smith, L.R.D. Brynildson, H.F. Flanigan, J.G. Gray, D. Spurlock

University of New Mexico School of Medicine, Albuquerque, N.Mex.;
Medical College of Georgia, Augusta, Ga., USA

Key Words. Computer · Stereotactic surgery · Brain mapping · Computerized atlas maps · Thalamus · Electrophysiological maps

Abstract. A computerized anatomic atlas mapping technique has been developed and used to determine target sites for stereotactic thalamotomies. The digitized stereotactic atlases of Schaltenbrand and Bailey, Van Buren and Borke, and Schaltenbrand and Wahren are used in conjunction with an associated electrophysiological data base to determine the intended target site on MR images of the diencephalon. This mapping technique uses the 'Brierley and Beck' proportional hypothesis for thalamic nuclear determination. Target site determination by this method was found to be very accurate, and frequently the mere placement of the probe in the target site resulted in tremor cessation.

Historically, the ventralis intermedius (VIM) nucleus of the thalamus has been the target site of choice for alleviation of tremor with some authors focusing the lesion site at the basal portion of VIM in the dorsal subthalamic area [1, 2]. Brierley and Beck [1] hypothesized that the thalamic nuclei appear to occupy relatively constant proportions of the entire thalamic length. Newer imaging techniques for stereotaxy, including MRI annd CT [3, 4], allow direct visualization of the total thalamic length in various dimensions. Thus, we hypothesize that MR computer-enhanced images of the diencephalon used in conjunction with scaled stereotactic anatomic map overlays and computer-sorted electrophysiological responses from a diencephalic stimulation and recording data base can define thalamic nuclear regions and be used to optimize target localization for dyskinesia.

1011–6125/92/0584–0030 $ 2.75/0

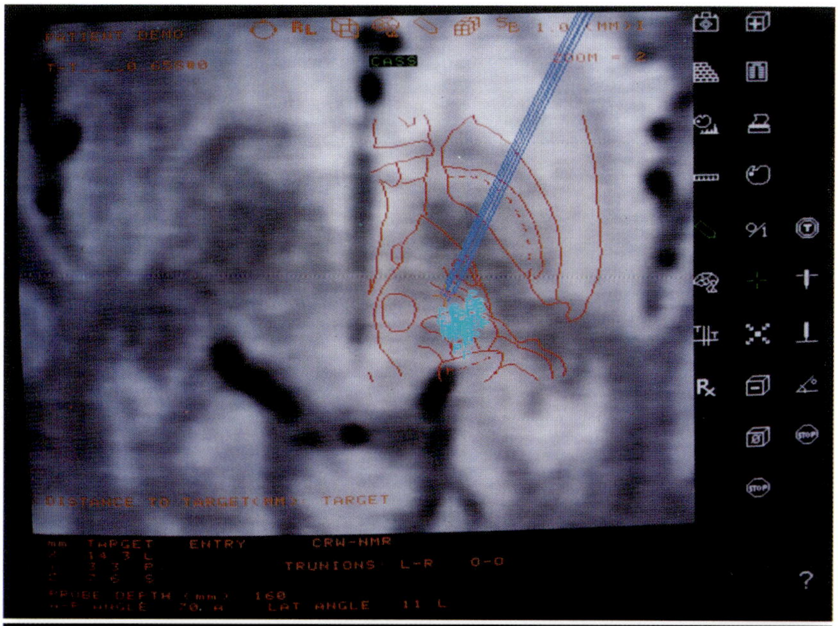
PATIENT DEMO
CASS
ZOOM = 2
DISTANCE TO TARGET(MM): TARGET
mm TARGET ENTRY CRW-NMR
TRUNIONS L-R 0-0
PROBE DEPTH (mm) 160
A-P ANGLE 70 A LAT ANGLE 11 L
?

1

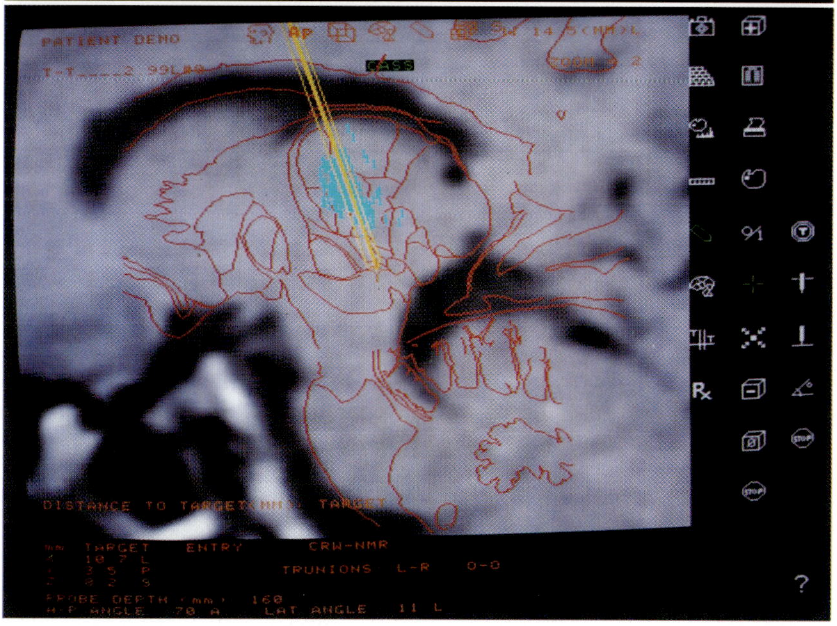
PATIENT DEMO
AP
CASS
DISTANCE TO TARGET(MM): TARGET
mm TARGET ENTRY CRW-NMR
TRUNIONS L-R 0-0
PROBE DEPTH (mm) 160
A-P ANGLE 70 A LAT ANGLE 11 L
?

2

Fig. 1. Horizontal MR image showing composite map from Schaltenbrand and Bailey at the level of the intercommissural plane. Map has been fitted to patient's brain dimensions. Electrophysiological data showing touch-evoked responses for face are shown in the region of the main sensory nucleus (blue cluster of responses in ventralis caudalis). Stereotactic probe is simulated for a target anterior to these responses with its tip in the dorsal subthalamic region. Note stereotactic frame coordinates for target and probe's trajectory.

Fig. 2. Sagittal MR image with atlas map from Schaltenbrand and Wahren [6] tailored to brain dimensions. Electrophysiological responses showing nonevoked rhythmic microelectrode recording units in the region of VIM (blue cluster of responses). Stereotactic probe's trajectory is simulated through this cluster of responses with its tip in the target area of the dorsal subthalamus.

The accuracy of MRI for any stereotactic or mapping technique must be considered. Although MRI in various views has greatly enhanced the ability to discern anatomic structures in the brain, its limitations have been due to errors induced by distortions inherent in the scanning technique and stereotactic frame design. For our method of stereotactic MRI and anatomic atlas mapping, we have used MRI scanning parameters with limited spin-echo in conjunction with a saline-filled stereotactic frame fiducial localization system which has been found to produce little distortion in MR images. Thin slices of 1.5 mm or less reduce errors due to volume averaging. A computer program which has been designed to detect any significant image distortion beyond a given tolerance level is used with this stereotactic imaging and mapping technique. In addition, simultaneous target determination on frontal, sagittal and horizontal MR images increases the accuracy of this imaging technique.

The digitized stereotactic atlases of Schaltenbrand and Bailey [5], Schaltenbrand and Wahren [6], and Van Buren and Borke [7] are used in conjunction with an electrophysiological data base [3–4] for individually selecting intended target sites. Such digital atlas maps and electrophysiological data can be scaled and superimposed on the patient's actual MR images (fig. 1, 2) to proportion thalamic nuclei according to the Brierley and Beck [1] proportional hypothesis for thalamic nuclear positions. In a recent small series of 8 cases, the dorsal subthalamic region with the stereotactic probe's trajectory through the sagittal length of VIM was used as the optimal target site for dyskinesias. Target site position was confirmed by a microstimulation technique using a side extruding electrode [2–4]. This mapping method and target site localization and trajectory were found to be very accurate in relieving dyskinetic movements. As previously noted by Bertrand et al. [2], the mere placement of the probe in the target site resulted in tremor cessation. This imaging and mapping technique, with neurophysiological confirmation, is proposed as a means of optimizing the initial target determinations for dyskinesias.

References

1 Brierley JB, Beck E: The significance in human stereotactic brain surgery of individual variation in the diencephalon and globus pallidus. J Neurol Neurosurg Psychiatry 1959;22:287–298.

2 Bertrand C, Martinez SN, Hardy J, Molina-Negro P, Velasco F: Stereotactic Surgery for Parkinsonism. Prog Neurol Surg 1973;79–112.
3 Hardy TL: Stereotactic CT atlases; in Lunsford LD (ed): Modern Stereotactic Surgery. Boston, Nijhoff, 1988, chapt 34.
4 Hardy TL: A method for MRI and CT mapping of diencephalic somatotopography. Stereotact Funct Neurosurg 1989;52:242–249.
5 Schaltenbrand G, Bailey P: Introduction to Stereotaxis with an Atlas of the Human Brain. New York, Thieme, 1959.
6 Schaltenbrand G, Wahren W: Atlas for Stereotaxy of the Human Brain, ed 2. Stuttgart, Thieme, 1977.
7 Van Buren JM, Borke RC: Variations and Connections of the Human Thalamus. New York, Springer, 1972, vol 1 and 2.

T.L Hardy, MD, Neurosurgery Department, Lovelace Medical Center,
5400 Blvd. SE, Albuquerque, NM 87108 (USA)

Proceedings of the Meeting of the American Society for Stereotactic and Functional Neurosurgery, Pittsburgh, Pa., June 16–19, 1991
Stereotact Funct Neurosurg 1992;58:33–38

Application of Magnetic Resonance Imaging in Functional Stereotactic Thalamotomy for the Evaluation of Individual Variations of the Thalamus

Y. Kawashima, H.J. Chen, A. Takahashi, M. Hirato, C. Ohye
Department of Neurosurgery, Gunma University, Gunma, Japan

Key Words. Stereotactic surgery · Thalamotomy · Human thalamus · MRI

Abstract. An application of MRI in functional stereotactic thalamotomy is presented. To estimate the individual anatomic variations of the thalamus prior to stereotactic thalamotomy, a special study using a proton density image that shows myeloarchitectonic features of the thalamus was performed. The proton density MRI was demonstrated to be very useful to determine the safest trajectory and tentative target point. However, as a detailed functional localization of the thalamic subnuclei cannot be yet obtained by MRI, the final target should be decided on the basis of electrophysiological findings.

Stereotactic thalamotomy has been performed as a therapeutic procedure for parkinsonian tremor and rigidity as well as for other involuntary movement disorders and central pain syndrome. The final placement of the radiofrequency therapeutic lesion should be decided by considering the individual antomic and functional differences of the thalamus. For this purpose, we rely on the electrophysiological findings obtained by depth microelectrode recording. The optimal radiofrequency target to ameliorate various kinds of tremor is the most lateral part of the ventral intermediate (VIM) nucleus where the kinesthetic neurons and/or tremor time-locked rhythmic discharges are recorded [1, 2]. However, in order to get the intended electrophysiological findings, an accurate orientation of the recording electrode toward the tentative target based on a neuroradiological study is essential. In this re-

1011–6125/92/0584–0033 $ 2.75/0

port, we present the characteristic MRI features of the thalamus and our strategy for the application of MRI in functional stereotactic thalamotomy.

Clinical Material and Methods

25 patients with Parkinson's disease (15 male, 10 female; age range 34–75 years) and 10 patient with essential tremor (8 male, 2 female; age range, 39–63 years) underwent preoperative MRI studies.

MRI was performed by using a 1.5-tesla MRI unit (Magnetom, Siemens Medical System). Proton density axial images (TR2000-Te19), nearly parallel to the intercommissural line (IC line), and oblique images parallel to the intraoperative trajectory, about 45° to the IC line, were taken. The axial images were taken with 3 mm slice thickness and 3.6 mm interslice interval. The oblique images were taken at 4 mm slice thickness and 5 mm interslice interval.

The width of the third ventricle and the distance from the midline to the thalamocapsular border were measured on the oblique image that contained the intraoperative elctrode trajectory, namely the image passing 5 mm anterior to the posterior commissure (PC). During the operation, ventriculography was performed and electrode coordinates were calcualted based on the PC and IC line. The lateral coordinate was determined by considering the thalamocapsular border shown on MRI. The final target for the radiofrequency thalamic lesion was determined by electrophysiological findings using a depth microelectrode [2].

Results

Compared with T_1- or T_2-weighted images, the proton density image was found to be the most suitable image to distinguish deep cerebral structures. In the proton density image, the medial, dorsal and caudal parts of the thalamus are shown as high-signal intensity zones, while the ventrolateral part of the thalamus, namely the ventral nuclear group, is shown as a slightly low-signal intensity zone compared to other nuclear groups in the thalamus (fig. 1). These findings are strikingly similar to and compatible with the myeloarchitectonic features of Schaltenbrand and Wahren's atlas [3]. The nerve fibers are sparse in the medial, dorsal and caudal parts of the thalamus, compared to the fiber-rich ventral nuclear group. The ventral nuclear group is subdivided into lateropolaris, ventrooralis, VIM and ventrocaudalis nuclei based on their characteristic features of their cellular and fibrous components [4]. Although these subnuclei cannot be distinguished on to-

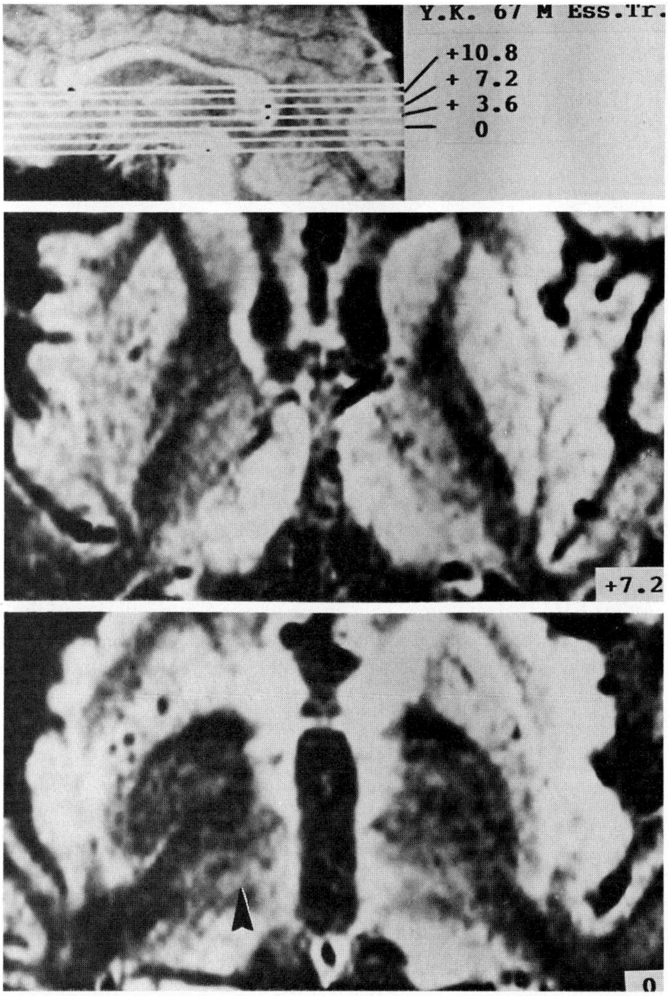

Fig. 1. Selected examples of proton density axial images (TR2000-TE19), nearly parallel to the IC line. The number indicated on each image represents the level of each image. The ventrolateral part of the thalamus is shown as a slightly low-signal intensity zone contrasting with other nuclear groups in the thalamus. The VCPC nucleus is visible as a high-signal intense small area (arrow).

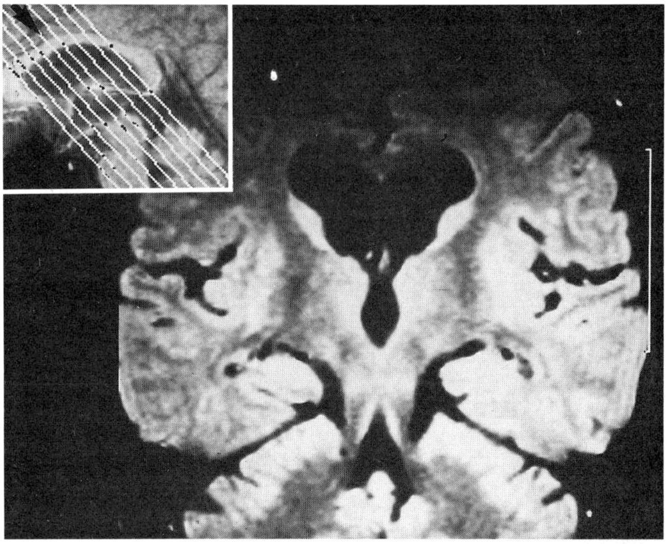

Fig. 2. Proton density oblique image that coincides with the intraoperative electrode trajectory for VIM thalamotomy. This image passes 5 mm anterior to the PC at an angle of about 45° to the IC line. On this image, we can clearly see he fiber bundle from the cerebellum going up to the lateral part of the ventral thalamus after crossing at the cerebellar decussation.

day's MR images, careful observation will reveal the ventrocaudalis parvocellularis nucleus (VCPC). As shown in figure 1, the VCPC is visible as a high-signal intense small area surrounded by a low-signal myelin-rich area, at about the level of the IC line or lower. It is interesting to note that myeloarchitecturally the VCPC internus is clearly separable as it lacks a definite myelin feltwork [5].

The MR image parallel to the intraoperative oblique trajectory is also practically informative. For example, an oblique MR image which may coincide with an intraoperative trajectory is made passing 5 mm anterior to the PC (as the tentative target point for VIM thalamotomy is placed 5 mm anterior to the PC, on the IC line), at about an angle of 45° to the IC line. On this image, we can clearly see the fiber bundle from the cerebellum going up to the lateral part of the ventral thalamus after crossing at the cerebellar decussation (fig. 2).

On MR images, the distance from the tentative target point to various subcortical structures, such as the caudate nucleus and border of the thalamus, along the intended trajectory could be measured before operation. The findings of the depth electrode recording during operation corresponded well with the anatomic findings depicted on MRI.

The width of the third ventricle and the distance from the midline to the thalmocapsular border measured on the MR image containing the electrode trajectory correlated well. In our cases, it was 18.8 ± 1.4 mm in women and 20.5 ± 1.2 mm in men. Even in cases with the same third ventricular width, 4- to 5-mm differences were found in the distance from the midline to the thalamocapsular border. There were no significant differences between parkinsonian cases and cases with essential tremor.

We determined the lateral coordinate of the electrode depending on MRI. In cases with the usual thalamocapsular border, about 20 mm from the midline, we took 16–17 mm as lateral coordinate, namely 3–4 mm medial to the thalamocapsular border. Thus, we could find kinesthetic neurons and/or tremor time-locked discharge in all cases. Finally, a small coagulation (40–60 mm^3) at this site could abolish the contralateral tremor without any undesirable neurological deficit.

The radiofrequency lesions that ameliorate tremor were verified to be located in the ventrolateral part of the thalamus just medial to the internal capsule postoperatively.

Discussion

Proton density images show the myeloarchitectonic features of the thalamus. The signal intensity of the ventral nuclear group is lower than that of other thalamic nuclear groups.

The common target for various types of tremor is considered to be the most lateral part of the VIM nucleus, where the kinesthetic neurons distribute [1, 2]. The target is located just medial to the internal capsule, and careful operative planning is necessary. Evaluation of the thalamocapsular border is essential for safe setting of the tentative target point. Prior to MRI becoming available, the lateral coordinate of the target was determined by considering the width of the third ventricle on ventriculography or CT. In cases with enlarged third ventricle, the tentative target point was placed 1–2 mm more lateral than in cases with a normally sized ventricle. Now we are able to estimate exactly the thalamocapsular border of each patient by MRI.

To get excellent and constant operative results, MRI is very useful. However, MRI does not show a functitonal localization of the thalamus and, therefore, the final radiofrequency lesion should be made on the basis of electrophysiological findings.

References

1 Ohye C, Schibazaki T, Hirato M, Kawashima Y, Matsumara M: Strategy of selective VIM thalamotomy guided by microrecording. Stereotact Funct Neurosurg 1990;54/55:186–191.
2 Ohye C: Selective thalamotomy for movement disorders: Microrecording stimulation techniques and results; in Lunsford LD (ed): Modern Stereotactic Neurosurgery. Boston, Nijhoff, 1988, pp 315–331.
3 Schaltenbrand G, Wahren W: Atlas for Sterotaxy of Human Brain. Stuttgart, Thieme, 1977.
4 Ohye C: Thalamus; in Paxinos G (ed): The Human Nervous System. New York, Academic Press, 1990, pp 439–468.
5 Hassler R: Architectonic organization of the thalamic nuclei; in Schaltenbrand G, Walker AE (eds): Stereotaxy of Human Brain, ed 2. Stuttgart, Thieme, 1982, pp 140–180.

Dr. Y. Kawashima, Department of Neurosugery, Gunma University, 3-39-22, Showa-machi, Maebashi, Gunma (Japan)

Proceedings of the Meeting of the American Society for Stereotactic and Functional Neurosurgery, Pittsburgh, Pa., June 16–19, 1991
Stereotact Funct Neurosurg 1992;58:39–44

Neurophysiological Atlas Created by Mapping of Clinical Responses Elicited on Electrical Stimulation of the Human Thalamus

Masafumi Yoshida

Department of Neurosurgery, Kurume University School of Medicine, Kurume, Japan

Key Words. Computer · Data processing · Functional atlas · Neurophysiology · Parkinsonism · Schaltenbrand-Bailey's atlas · Stereotactic surgery · Thalamus

Abstract. By computer processing of intraoperative neurophysiological data and intraoperative X-ray films, and using a 0.5-mm-step three-dimensional atlas created by interpolation of Schaltenbrand-Bailey's atlas, a neurophysiological atlas based on clinical responses upon electrical stimulation of the subcortical structures of patients who underwent stereotactic surgery in the awake state was created. There was considerable overlap in the distribution of motor and sensory responses in the vicinity of the ventral intermediate (VIM) thalamus: however, motor responses, particularly irregular movements, tended to be confined within the VIM and ventro-oralis posterior (VOP), whereas sensory responses tended to be localized in the VIM and ventroposterolateral nuclei, with considerable extension into the ventroposterior subthalamic region. In either motor or sensory responses, no definite somatotopic pattern could be determined.

During stereotactic procedures, a voluminous amount of neurophysiological data can be obtained from patients in the awake state. These data are precisely correlated to a point defined on a three-dimensional coordinate system and can be referred to anatomic structures by use of a standard anatomic atlas based on the same coordinate system. Therefore, by plotting these intraoperative data together with an anatomic atlas, a functional atlas can be created and the functional organization in relation to the anatomic structure can be elucidated. In this respect, the 0.5-mm-step three-dimensional atlas [1] created by interpolation of Schaltenbrand-Bailey's atlas [2] has the advantage in that any point on the three-dimensional coordinate system can be plot-

1011–6125/92/0584–0039 $ 2.75/0

ted on an atlas which is within 0.25 mm from that particular point, and that by serial display of the various sections of the atlas with desired angulation and rotation the three-dimensional anatomic (or, functional, in case of a functional atlas) organization can be more clearly illustrated.

In this presentation a computer-processed functional atlas based on clinical responses upon electrical stimulation of human subcortical structues is presented, and the functional organization of the thalamus and adjacent structures is briefly discussed.

Clinical Material and Methods

The clinical material consisted of 19 parkinsonian patients and 3 patients with tremor and thalamic or pseudothalamic pain, respectively. They underwent a total number of 29 stereotactic procedures. Various target areas, primarily in and around the thalamus ventro-oralis posterior (VOP) and ventral intermediate (VIM) nuclei for parkinsonism and tremor, posterior limb of the internal capsule and ventroposterolateral (VPL) nucleus for deafferentation pain syndrome] were approached via frontal burr holes. For each stereotactic procedure, 1–3 trajectories were explored and, for each trajectory, a 3- to 5-mm-step stimulation study was performed at several points in the vicinity of the target area with the use of a bipolar, coaxial (stainless steel or tungsten) semi-microelectrode whose tip diameter is approximately 50 μm. Stimulation parameters were 2 mA constant current square wave with frequency ranging from 5 to 90 Hz and pulse width from 0.1 to 0.5 ms.

For calculation of coordinates of stimulation points, intraoperative X-ray films visualizing cerebral reference points and location of stimulation electrodes were digitized. By programing, the computer will calculate three-dimensional coordinates of stimulation points when simply given the depth (the distance from the target) of the advancing electrode along a trajectory. In this process, parallax and magnification, as well as tilt and rotation of the patients' head, were all corrected. Modality and somatic representation of clinical responses upon elctrical stimulation of subcortical structures were coded, computer-processed and displayed together with the three-dimensional atlas. Stimulation responses were grouped into three modality categories, i.e. sensory, motor and emotional or autonomic, and analyzed.

Results

Since, in all cases, subcortical targets were approached via frontal burr holes and, in the majority of cases, VIM was targeted, the anatomic distribution of stimulation points converged in the ventrolateral portion of the VIM and VOP area with considerable divergence in both

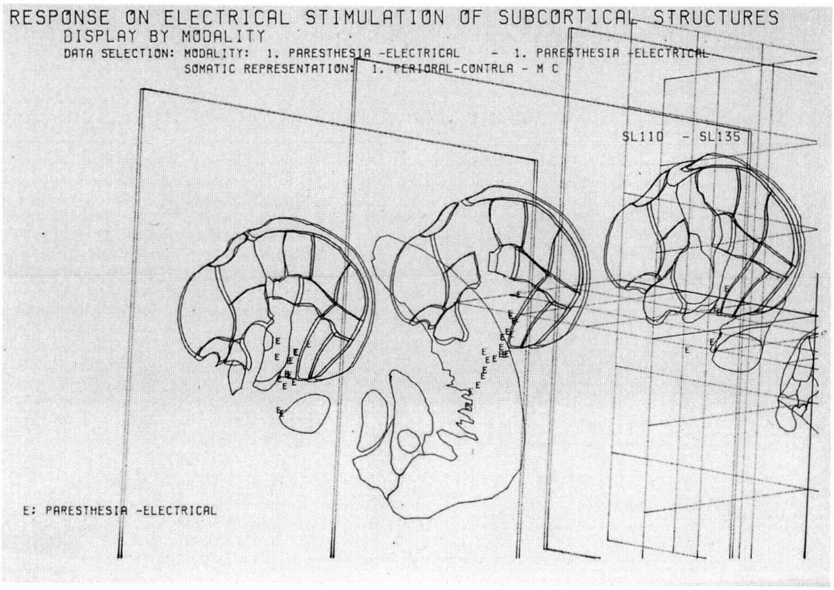

Fig. 1. Sensory responses. Paresthesia of electrical sensation. This response modality is coded as 'E' and plotted at stimulation sites. Display range = Sl. 110–135.

the anterodorsolateral and posteroventromedial direction from the VIM.

Sensory Responses (fig. 1). The majority of responses were paresthesias of electrical sensation, and there were a few instances of paresthesias of tingling, warm and cold sensation. The stimulation points which elicited sensory responses were located in the lateral portion of the VIM and VPL, but also extended considerably ventroposteromedially into the subthalamic area. When the somatic representation of the sensory responses LS examined, the majority represented the face, hand or upper extremity region. In only a few instances was the lower limb represented, and there does not seem to exist any apparent somatotopic distribution.

Motor Responses (fig. 2). Except perhaps for irregular movement, no pure motor response was noted, but many were recognized in relation to tremor. Therefore, a motor response can probably be subcategorized into those related to tremor, i.e. arrest, suppression and en-

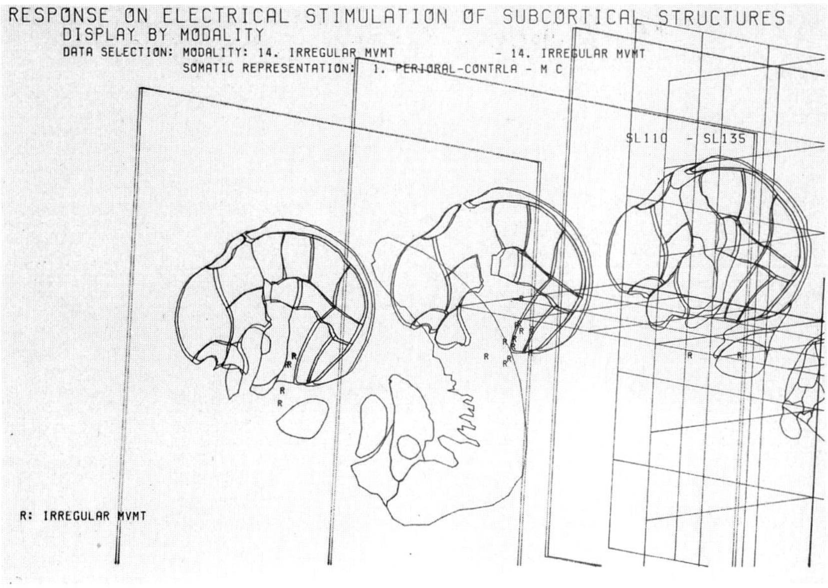

Fig. 2. Motor responses. Irregular movement. This response modality is coded as 'R' and plotted at stimulation sites. Display range = Sl. 110–135.

hancement of tremor, and those independent of tremulous movement, i.e. irregular movement of upper limbs. Regardless of subcategories, the motor responses were primarily elicited in the VOP and VIM. There was some extension posteroventrally into the subthalamic area, particularly of tremor-related responses. Irregular movement was more characteristically and distinctly localized in the lateral portion of the VOP and VIM than any other subcategory. When somatic representation was examined, they were exclusively noted in the upper limb and especially in the hand region.

Emotional, Autonomic and Other Responses. Responses of this category, some of which were difficult to classify, were elicited upon stimulation of rather wide areas, but many were primarily noted in the subthalamic field or in the upper midbrain.

Discussion

Advantages of this kind of study are that neurophysiological data obtained are from the human brain in an awake state, and that data-obtaining points are precisely located on a three-dimensional coordinate system and therefore can be correlated to a standard anatomic atlas.

On the other hand, disadvantages, which primarily stem from the fact that this is a clinical study performed during a treatment-oriented invasive procedure, and therefore freedom of choice of exploration sites or trajectory location, patient population, data acquisition time and modality for neurophysiological studies, are all limited. Certainly no control data of this kind from humans without pathology are available.

Even with these limitations, the neurophysiological atlas in and around the thalamus presented in this study showed a fairly characteristic distribution pattern for each of the various response modalities, indicating the presence of a neurophysiologically distinct functional system in relation to anatomic substates. The overlap in distribution of sensory and motor responses in the vicinity of VIM probably indicates the importance of this subnucleus in integrating the sensory and motor systems and for coordinated motor control.

In either sensory or motor responses, no apparent somatotopic pattern was noted within the thalamus or in the internal capsule. Since somatotopy in these areas may be critically influenced by individual anatomic variation which is probably related to the size of the third ventricle, and the location of the thalamocapsular border and ventral border of the thalamus, detailed study integrating these parameters will be necessary before conclusions can be drawn.

The computer data-processing system used in this study is capable of handling any three-dimensional data which can be reformatted to be aligned to the anterior/posterior-commissure-based three-dimensional coordinate system. Such data include anatomic data from CT and MRI and functional data from PET. Therefore, when these data, as well as other intraoperative neurophysiological data such as general neuronal activity (neural noise) [3] and evoked potentials, are integrated into this system, more detailed and comprehensive delineation of the functional organization of subcortical structures might be possible.

References

1 Yoshida M: Creation of a three-dimensional atlas by interpolation from Schaltenbrand-Bailey's atlas. Appl Neurophysiol 1987;50:45–48.
2 Schaltenbrand G, Bailey P (eds): Introduction to Stereotaxis with an Atlas of Human Brain. Stuttgart, Thieme, 1959.
3 Yoshida M, Kuramoto S: Neural noise as a real time guide for tumor site localization during stereotactic biopsy of brain tumors. Appl Neurophysiol 1987;50: 195–199.

Masafumi Yoshida, MD, Department of Neurosurgery,
Kurume University School of Medicine, 67 Asahi-machi, Kurume, 830 (Japan)

Proceedings of the Meeting of the American Society for Stereotactic and Functional Neurosurgery, Pittsburgh, Pa., June 16–19, 1991
Stereotact Funct Neurosurg 1992;58:45–51

A New Multimodality Correlative Imaging Technique for VOP/VIM (VL) Thalamotomy Procedures

Bruce A. Kall[a], *Stephan J. Goerss*[b], *Patrick J. Kelly*[b]

[a] Section of Patient Care Systems, and [b] Department of Neurologic Surgery, Mayo Clinic, Rochester, Minn., USA

Key Words. Functional Stereotaxis · Thalamotomy · Correlative imaging · Magnetic resonance imaging · Computerized tomography

Abstract. This paper describes our experience at Mayo Clinic with a new technique for planning ventro-oralis posterior (VOP) ventral intermediate (ventrolateral) VIM (VL) thalamotomy procedures for selected patients with medically intractable tremor. This new method employs a *multimodality correlative imaging technique* for determining the lesion target point on MR images. At surgery, stereotactic frame settings for the final lesion target were ultimately determined by stereotactic ventriculography modified by neurophysiological recording. Acceptable correlation was found between the multimodality correlative imaging method and the actual target coordinates determined by ventriculography and semi-microelectrode recording.

CT and MRI may be used to visualize the axial configuration of the third ventricle, thalamus and internal capsule for functional stereotactic procedures. Furthermore, the anterior (AC) and posterior (PC) commissures are easily visualized on sagittal MRI. Our group has developed a multimodality correlative imaging technique that utilizes transverse and sagittal MRI and axial CT images to plan a lesion location for VOP/ventral intermediate (ventrolateral) [VOP/VIM (VL)] thalamotomy procedures for patients with medically intractable tumor.

This technique is a variation of our previously reported techniques for correlating targets and volumes from CT and MRI [1, 2]. However, during surgery, the actual stereotactic frame settings used for the lesion site were calculated by stereotactic positive contrast ventriculog-

1011–6125/92/0584–0045 $ 2.75/0

raphy with the laterality modified by semi-microelectrode recording [3, 4]. Acceptable results were noted when ventriculography/neurophysiological recording technique.

Methods and Materials

Intrumentation and Data Acquisition

We employ the Compass Stereotactic System (Stereotactic Medical Systems, Rochester, Minn., USA) for stereotactic localization and targeting. Briefly, patients undergo stereotactic CT and MRI scanning with a relocatable stereotactic headframe applied under local anesthesia. CT scanning is performed on a General Electric 9800 unit which is used to collect 5-mm-thick images overlapping every 3 mm using a 34.5-cm field of view. A series of scans are also performed on a General Electric Sigma 1.5-tesla MRI unit using a 24-cm field of view. Three series are perfomed: (1) 4-mm-thick, adjacent TE20-TR5000 sagittal images; (2) TE 30/80-TR2000 4-mm-thick transverse images 5 mm apart, and (3) IR170-TR2000 5-mm-thick adjacent transverse images. All images are then transferred to the operating room computer and image system. These images are initially used to plan a target for the ventriculogram, which is performed in the operating room on the Compass three-dimensional positioner. The headframe is then removed and replaced on the day of surgery.

Computer and Imaging System

The computer and image system (Sun 4/300 workstation, Sun Microsystems, Mountain View, Calif., USA, and a Vicom VME image processor, Vicom Systems, Fremont, Calif., USA, drives a multimodality treatment-planning console consisting of 3 black-and-white and 1 color monitors and a CRT. All software was custom-developed using the C and Pascal programming languages.

Multimodality Correlative Imaging Technique

Our new multimodality correlative imaging technique employs sagittal and transverse MRI images and axial CT scans. All images in every series are initially localized by scanning for the position of the fiducial reference markers which are deposited on each image from a localization device that was applied to the headframe while each scan was performed. Each point on every image may then be translated into the x, y and z coordinate system of the Compass three-dimensional positioner. This allows automatic computer determination of correlating points between modalities and planes [1, 2].

Two sagittal midline slices are selected from the MRI series: one to localize the position of the AC and PC, and one to measure the height of the thalamus. The surgeon selects the position of AC and PC by moving a cursor over the midline image so that each point is noted (fig. 1). The computer determines the plane of AC-PC and locates its midpoint. A perpendicular is erected from the midpoint of the AC-PC plane and translated onto an appropriate lateral sagittal image showing the body of the thalamus. A point at the superior aspect of the thalamus on the perpendicular is selected, and the thalamic height is measured and is then transferred back onto the midline image.

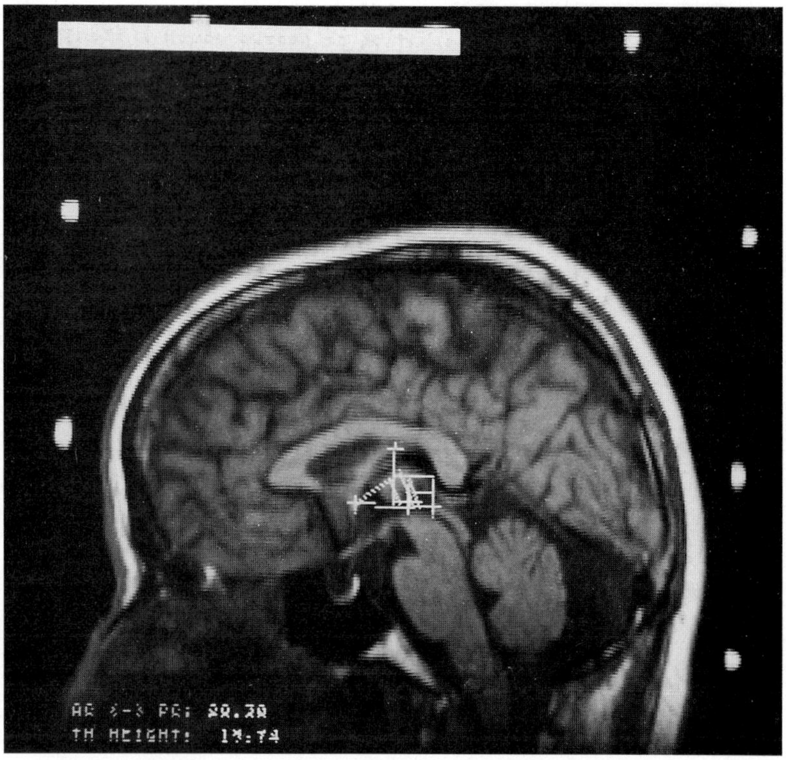

Fig. 1. Midline sagittal MR image with the location of AC and PC, AC-PC plane, perpendicular from its midpoint, and location on superior aspect of thalamus noted. The subnuclear divisions of the lateral ventral nuclear masses of the thalamus are displayed and the surgeon selects a location (large cursor) 1 mm anterior to the junction of VOP and VIM approximately 2.5 mm above AC-PC in the posterior portion of VOP.

Our software then scales and draws the subnuclear divisions of the lateral ventral nuclear masses of the thalamus (on the image showing AC and PC) by computerization of a method developed for positive contrast ventriculography originally proposed by Talairach and modified by Guiot. A point is then selected by the physician using the cursor that is 1 mm anterior to the junction of VOP and VIM approximately 2.5 mm above the AC-PC plane in the posterior portion of VOP. A three-dimensional coordinate is then calculated for this point and is automatically correlated to the closest pixel on the closest axial CT image. A line is then drawn through this point parallel to the midline on the CT image and the surgeon selects a point on this line on the lateral wall of the third ventricle. A point 11.5 mm lateral to this point (in the appropriate hemi-

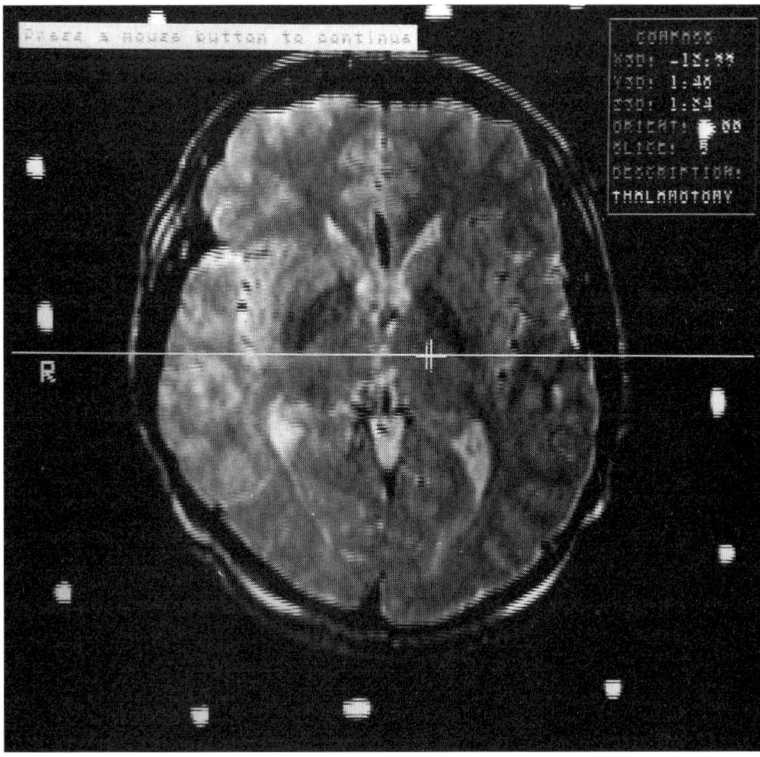

Fig. 2. Transverse MR image with line through point correlated from CT 11.5 mm lateral to a point on the lateral aspect of the third ventricle. The final proposed location for the lesion location is then selected on this line by the physician (large cursor), and the x, y, z Compass frame settings are calculated and displayed.

sphere for the procedure) is then calculated and displayed by the computer. This CT-derived coordinate 11.5 mm lateral to the third ventricle is then automatically correlated to a point on a slice from either of the transverse MRI series that best shows the internal capsule (fig. 2). A line parallel to the midline through this correlated point is drawn and the surgeon selects the proposed target location for the lesion in the midlateral portion of VOP. The stereotactic coordinates of this point are then calculated (x_{3d}, y_{3d}, z_{3d}) and compared to the ventriculography modified by neurophysiological recording coordinate. The time required to perform all of the above operations and determine the final target point is approximately 1 min.

Table 1. Comparison between the ventriculography modified by neurophysiological recording (VMNR) and the multimodality correlative imaging technique (MCIT)

Patient	VMNR			MCIT			Δx	Δy	Δz	3 D dist.
	x	y	z	x	y	z				
1	–11.70	4.50	6.58	–11.20	6.27	8.20	–0.50	–1.77	–1.62	2.451
2	–16.88	4.66	17.24	–16.74	7.11	17.01	–0.14	–2.45	0.23	2.4648
3	–15.99	1.32	11.18	–16.98	4.44	13.69	0.99	–3.12	–2.51	4.1249
4	11.50	3.00	5.00	12.28	3.98	4.17	–0.78	–0.98	0.83	1.5026
5	–12.49	0.07	0.66	–12.99	1.48	1.24	0.50	–1.41	–0.58	1.6045
6	15.47	–0.36	1.20	14.75	0.84	2.60	0.72	–1.20	–1.40	1.9795
7	–12.63	1.83	10.08	–14.71	1.61	6.78	2.08	0.22	3.30	3.907
8	–16.75	4.05	18	–15.35	3.82	18.33	–1.40	0.23	–0.33	1.4566

Average errors: x, 0.89 mm; y, 1.42 mm; z, 1.35 mm; 3D, 2.58 mm.

Ventriculography and Microelectrode Recording

Our group has continued to use positive contrast ventriculography for stereotactic thalamotomies, despite the availability of CT and MRI scanning. A stereotactic ventriculogram is performed with the patient in the stereotactic headholder on the Compass positioner. This is usually performed on the same day as CT and MRI data acquisition.

The stereotactic y coordinate is calculated from a point 1 mm anterior to the anterior border of VIM while the z coordinate is calculated from a point 2.5 mm above AC-PC. The x coordinate (laterality) is confirmed by semi-microelectrode recording. The trajectory of the microelectrode recording is directed from the stereotactic frame and passes through the ventralis caudalis externus (VCE) to a point 1 mm anterior to PC, initially 11.5 mm lateral to the lateral wall of the third ventricle on the AC-PC line. The final laterality in VOP/VIM is determined from the somatotopy of the evoked responses [4]. In general the correct laterality of the target site in VOP/VIM for upper extremity tremor corresponds to the laterality of the thumb and index finger in VCE.

Results

A reasonable correlation was found comparing the x, y, z stereotactic coordinates from the multimodality correlative imaging method and the ventriculography modified by neurophysiological recording method. The results for 8 patients are summarized in table 1.

Small differences were noted between the two techniques with not discernable pattern. Differences in x ranged from –0.14 mm in patient 2 to 2.08 mm in patient 7 with an average of 0.89 mm. The y errors were between 0.22 mm in patient 7 to –3.12 mm in patient 3, averaging 1.42 mm. The average error in z was 1.35 mm ranging in values from 0.23 mm in patient 2 to 3.30 mm in patient 7. The z error could be attributed to the slice thickness of the CT and MR images which varied from 4 to 5 mm. Each pixel on a CT and MR image is 0.673 and 0.937 mm respectively. Therefore, every pixel variation in selecting points on the CT of MRI could vary the results by close to 1 mm.

Discussion

The new multimodality correlative image technique described in the paper is a variation of calculation and correlation of target points from CT and MRI built-in to the Compass Stereotactic System. We have shown, in most cases, that target calculations performed using this new technique correlate well with actual frame coordinates used for the anatomic lesion derived from ventriculography modified by neurophysiological recording. Target coordinates derived by this new multimodality correlative image technique may become closer to those determined by the ventriculography/microelectrode method as digital radiological imaging resolution and spatial accuracy increases in the future. Nonetheless, stereotactic thalamotomy is a physiological procedure in addition to an anatomically based procedure. We feel that, irrespective of the method used for anatomic target coordinate determination, some method for physiological target corroboration should be employed in all patients undergoing VL thalamotomy for movement disorders.

Acknowledgements

Special acknowledgement is given to Ms. Cathy Hunt for helping in the collection and tabulation of coordinates and to Mr. Scott Stiving for software suggestions used in the multimodality correlation technique.

References

1 Kall BA, Kelly PJ, Goerss SJ, Earnest F IV: Cross-registration of point and lesion volumes from MR and CT. Proc 7th Annu Meet of Frontiers of Engineering and Computing in Health Care, 1985, pp 692–695.

2 Kelly PJ, Daumas-Duport C, Scheithauer T, Kall BA, Kispert DB: Stereotactic histological correlation of computed tomography and magnetic resonance imaging-defined abnormalities in patient with glial neoplasm. Mayo Clin Proc 1987;62: 450–459.

3 Kelly PJ: Microelectrode recording for the somatotopic placement of stereotactic thalamic lesions in the treatment of parkinsonian and cerebellar tremor. Appl Neurophysiol 1980;43:262–266.

4 Kelly PJ, Ahlskog JE, Goerss SJ, Daube JR, Duffy JR, Kall BA: Computer-assisted stereotactic ventralis lateralis thalamotomy with microelectrode recording control in patients with Parkinson's disease. Mayo Clin Proc 1987;62:655–664.

Bruce A. Kall, MS, Section of Patient Care Systems, Mayo Clinic,
200 First ST SW, 5-222, Rochester, MN 55095 (USA)

Proceedings of the Meeting of the American Society for Stereotactic and Functional Neurosurgery, Pittsburgh, Pa., June 16–19, 1991
Stereotactic Funct Neurosurg 1992;58:52–58

Spinal Cord Stimulation for Multiple Sclerosis: Quantifiable Benefits

Ross Davis, Sandra E. Emmonds

Section of Neurosurgery, Veterans Administration Medical Center and Kennebec Valley Medical Center, Augusta, Me., USA

Key Words. Spinal cord stimulation · Multiple sclerosis · Paraparesis · Quadriparesis

Abstract. From 1984 to 1991, a quantitative study of 5 multiple sclerosis (MS) patients has been determining benefits from epidural (C7–T1 level) spinal cord stimulation (SCS). The 5 patients (4 male, 1 female; 4 tetraparetics, 1 hemiparetic) were 36–45 years of age having had symptoms for 12–22 years. Five quantitative tests were given prior to and during SCS on 4–8 occasions; 'off' periods were planned and also did occur when the electrode(s) broke (3 patients). With SCS, hand dynamometry showed a 2- to 4-fold increase in the 3 patients with weak hand function. Jebson Hand Time Testing showed a rapidity improvement to 1/2–1/7 of time in the same 3 patients. Minnesota Manipulation Testing with SCS was improved to 1/3–1/2 of time in 2 of these 3 patients tested. Manual muscle strength increased in all patients by 20–50% in 'normal range'. Ambulation in the parallel bars increased with SCS in 2 of the 4 wheelchair patients, while the hemiparetic patient could walk without his cane. All patients showed varying quantifiable improvements with SCS, but over the duration of testing the patients slowly deteriorated. SCS is a rehabilitation option for the weakened MS patient, to be used earlier rather than later in the deterioration of MS patients.

Introduction

There have been 4 major reviews [1–4] in the last 10 years concerning the improvements of multiple sclerosis (MS) patients from spinal cord stimulation (SCS). Siegfried et al. [1] reviewed the literature from its initiation in 1973 to 1980 where 616 MS patients had been reported on, from which they culled 355 having had comprehensive evaluations with 200 (56%) improved. Bladder function improvements were seen in

1011–6125/92/0584–0052 $ 2.75/0

50–75% of cases stimulated. Of their own 36 MS patients [1], 1 showed very good improvement, with 20 having good improvement, 13 fair and 2 no improvement.

In 1985, Gybels and Van Roost [3] reviewed 39 papers on the effects of SCS on dystonic and hyperkinetic disorders in 1,008 patients. Whereas SCS cannot prevent deterioration in progressive neurological disorders, the literature showed useful overall relief from disabilities including MS in 10–45% of the case. No conclusions could be drawn as to differences in results using cervical versus thoracic SCS. SCS appears to decrease excessive spinal reflex activity.

In 1987, Koulousakis et al. [5] quantitatively evaluated 12 MS patients for 4 years with no deterioration observed. Of the 4 tetraplegic MS patients, only 1, who had a slight increase in tonus and could walk with canes, noticed an improvement in standing and walking ability, as well as urinary function. Of the 8 paraplegic MS patients, 6 showed an improved life-style in regards to the modalities of walking, endurance and bladder functions. Waltz et al. [6] also in 1987, reported moderate to marked benefits in 63% of 91 MS patients with cervical SCS using a quadripolar electrode.

Following our report [7] in 1981 of 44 (64%) of 69 MS patients benefiting in ambulation from SCS, we have now studied 5 new MS patients with quantitative testing to help answer the question as to whether and when SCS is a valuable therapy in the MS rehabilitation process.

Method

From 1984 to 1991, a quantitative study of 5 MS patients has been determining benefits from dorsal epidural (C7–T1 level) SCS. The 5 patients (4 male, 1 female) were 36–45 years of age having had symptoms for 12–22 years and had been slowly deteriorating (table 1). Four were tetraparetic and used a wheelchair or electric cart, and 1 was hemiparetic and used a cane and brace.

Stimulators

The first 4 patients undervent a trial of 3–7 days of SCS with an inserted electrode (3 percutaneously, 1 laminotomy) placed dorsally at the cervicothoracic junction [8]. If they showed a quantifiable improvement the stimulators (see table 1 for equipment) were internalized under local anesthesia. The fifth patient showed motor strength improvement at the time of lead implantation so her stimulator was inserted. The 3 Medtronic 'Pisces-Quad' and 2 NeuroMed 'Quadripolar' percutaneously inserted electrodes broke at the spinous process area in 6–12 months; 2 of 3 patients requested and

Table 1. Detailed information and quantitative results of 5 MS patients following SCS – 1991

Patient information	Implant type age and date	Hand dynamometry
1. K.G. (DOB 8/38) 22 years of MS, tetraparesis L > R, 1987 wheelchair	Avery RF + Monolead, 45 years, 7/23/84; 1989 explanted and deterioration	tested 8×, 300% increase
2. M.P. (DOB 7/45) 14 years of MS, hemiparesis, used cane and brace	Medtronic Itrel, Resume SE-4 lead, 40 years, 6/27/86; explanted 4/18/91	tested 3×, 200% increase
3. T.B. (DOB 8/46) 12 years of MS, tetraparesis, 1986 wheelchair	Medtronic Itrel + Pisces-Quad, 40 years, 2/9/87; 2/88 no tingle, 2 months broken wire; 3/23/88 explanted and deterioration	tested 4×, 10–30% increase
4. A.D. (DOB 5/44) 15 years of MS, tetraparesis R > L, 1986 wheelchair	Medtronic Itrel + Pisces-Quad, 43 years, 5/20/87; 1/88 broken wire, 3/88 wire replaced; 1990 deterioration, 11/90 wire replaced; 1991 very weak, deteriorating, unable to be tested	tested 8×, 400% increase
5. C.T. (DOB 3/55) 14 years of MS, 1988 paraparesis to wheelchair	NeuroMed RF + Quad L, 33 years, 6/28/88; 12/19/88 broken wire replaced, 1/23/90 radioreceiver replaced, 1/91 broken wire and receiver replaced; very spastic paraplegic condition	tested 5×, no change

SCS: Avery Labs., Farmindale, N.Y., USA; Medtronic, Minneapolis, Minn., USA; NeuroMed, Ft. Lauderdale, Fla., USA. DOB = Date of birth; L = left; R = right.

received replacements. Two NeuroMed receivers failed at 6 and 12 months and were replaced. Three patients requested explantation after 5, 5 and 1 years, respectively, of SCS. Two patients continued to use their systems for 4 and 3 years from implantation (table 1). Stimulation pulse width and frequency were set at 200 μs and 30 pulses per second [8]; pulse amplitude was adjusted until the 'tingling' was comfortable.

Ambulation	Jebson Hand Time Testing	Minnesota Manipulation Time Testing	Manual muscle testing
tested 6×, 200–300% increase	tested 7×, improvement by 50%	tested 5×, improvement by 50%	tested 9×, 1.5–2× increase
7/86 no need for cane, 4/87 no need for brace	tested 6×, improvement by 50%	not tested	tested 5×, 2–3× increase
walked first time in 6 months	tested 2×, improvement by 25–30%	not tested	tested 3×, 1.2–3× increase
not applicable	tested 8×, improvement by 86%; able to make toys again	tested 7×, improvement by 50%	tested 6×, 2–3× increase
not applicable	tested 4×, no change	tested 3×, no change	tested 5×, 1.4× increase

Quantitative Testing

Five tests were performed prior to and during stimulation from 4 to 8 occasions by the physical and occupational therapists at the 2 medical centers involved. Attempts were made to have the same type of test done at the same time of day so the results would be comparable. The therapists were not told whether the stimulator was 'on' or 'off', although the patients could feel the stimulation paresthesias when on. Hand dynamometry measured hand grip in kilograms (table 1). Jebson Hand Time Testing was measured for fine and gross motor hand function in seconds. Minnesota Manipulation Time Testing was measured for their hand function in placing and turning blocks per second in a prespecified way. Manual muscle testing was done on all patients to measure their ability to move and hold a joint against gravity and maximum pressure; the resulting grade was converted to a percent of normal. Ambulation could only be tested on 3 patients – 2 holding onto parallel bars. Bladder function testing was attempted with cystometrograms (CMG) in 3 patients which showed preimplant low volume stimulation producing contractions interpreted as neurogenic bladders with spasms, plus outlet obstruction. The other 2 patients had symptomatic neurogenic bladders with urgency, retention and frequency. Two patients used catheterization. Although the study called for CMG testing on follow-up visits, it was done in only 1 patient because we found this testing difficult to arrange.

Results

Processed results from testing are seen in table 1. With SCS, hand dynamometry increased 2–4 times in the 3 patients with hand weakness and minimal to no increase in 2 patients with normal hand strength. Jebson Hand Time Testing showed an improvement by 1/2–1/7 of the time taken to complete the tasks in the same 3 patients, while minimal to no improvement was observed in the other 2 patients with almost normal hand function. Minnesota Manipulation Time Testing was reduced by 1/3–1/2 in 2 of the 2 patients with impaired hand function, while the patient with normal hand function showed no change. Manual muscle testing indicated an increase in weakened muscle in all 5 patients by 20–50% of 'normal' range. Ambulation improved in 1 patient who used an electric cart, while 1 patient was able to walk in the parallel bars for the first time in 6 months. A hemiparetic patient was able to leave off his brace and forego his cane with SCS. Only 1 of the patients had slight more bladder control.

Discussion

All 5 patients showed quantifiable improvements with SCS. The least assisted patient found most of her benefits in a decrease of spasticity and spasms, proven when the lead and receiver failed and was replaced. However, we have found during this 6-year study that the pa-

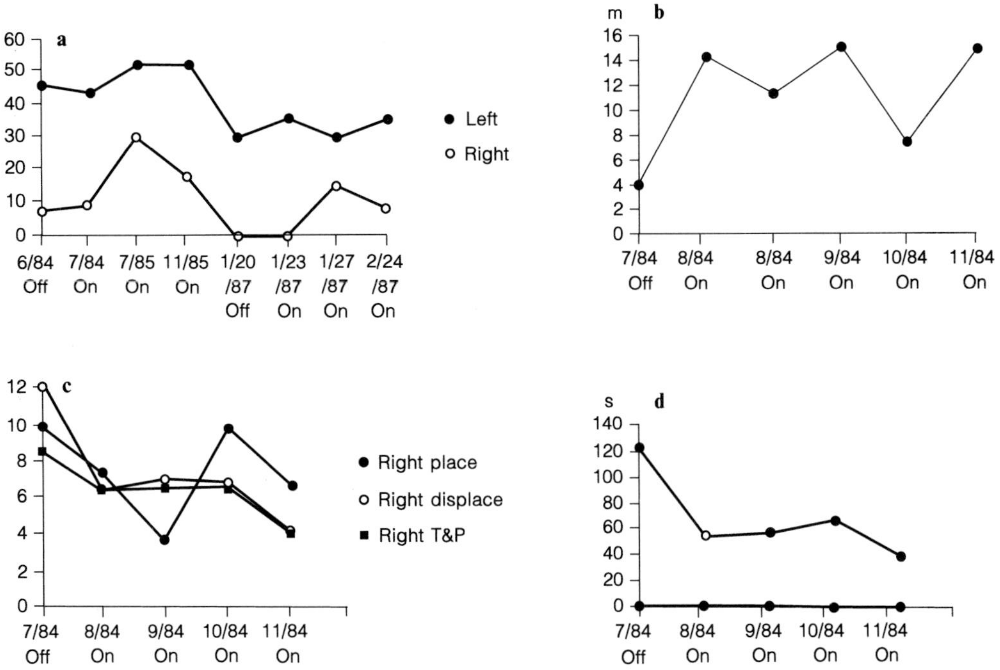

Fig. 1. a Hand dynamometry. **b** Ambulation in parallel bars. **c** Minnesota manipulation test. **d** Jebson: checkers right hand.

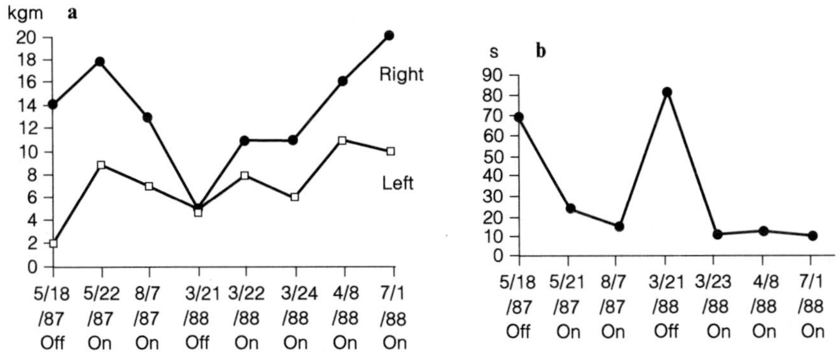

Fig. 2. a Hand dynamometry. **b** Jebson: checkers right hand.

tients continued to slowly deteriorate in their abilities and strength. The question raised is whether the long time use of SCS in MS is as effective as when first used, or is the MS process slowly causing the deterioration? The answer is most probably the latter as all 5 patients had been slowly deteriorating in their abilities and were in the 10–20+ year of the disease, when most neurological systems are affected [9]. No patient had had any remission in the previous year prior to SCS. When SCS was off, all abilities measuredly decreased until re-stimulated (fig. 1, 2). No patient had had a sudden deterioration or complication from the implant procedure or from SCS.

Prolonged SCS does appear to be a worthwhile and safe therapy for the rehabilitation program of the weakened MS patient, probably to be tested earlier rather than later, particularly as there now appears to be stronger electrodes and longer-lasting stimulators available.

References

1 Siegfried J, Lazorthes Y, Broggi G: Electrical spinal cord stimulation for spastic movement disorders. Appl Neurophysiol 1991;44:77–92.
2 Illis LS, Read DJ, Sedgwick EM, Tallis RC: Spinal cord stimulation in the United Kingdom. J Neurosurg Psychiatry 1983;46:299–230.
3 Gybels J, Van Roost D: Spinal cord stimulation for the modification of dystonic and hyperkinetic conditions: A critical review; in Eccles J, Dimitrijevic MR (eds): Recent Achievements in Restorative Neurology. Basel, Karger, 1985, pp 56–70.
4 Fredriksen TA, Bergmann S, Hesselberg JP, et al: Electrical stimulation in multiple sclerosis: Comparison of transcutaneous electrical stimulation and epidural spinal cord stimulation. Appl Neurophysiol 1986;49:4–24.
5 Koulousakis A, Buchhaas U, Nitter K: Application of SCS for movement disorders and spasticity. Acta Neurochir 1987(suppl 39):112–116.
6 Waltz JM, Andreesen WH, Hunt DP: Spinal cord stimulation and motor disorders. Pace 1987;10:180–204.
7 Davis R, Gray E, Kudzma J: Beneficial augmentation following dorsal column stimulation in some neurological diseases. Appl Neurophysiol 1981;44:37–49.
8 Davis R, Gray EF: Technical factors important to dorsal column stimulation. Appl Neurophysiol 1981;44:162–172.
9 Muller R: Studies in disseminated sclerosis. Acta Med Scand 1949(suppl 222):69.

Ross Davis, Section of Neurosurgery, Veterans Administration Medical Center and Kennebec Valley Medical Center, 55 Middle St., Augusta, ME 04330 (USA)

Proceedings of the Meeting of the American Society for Stereotactic and Functional Neurosurgery, Pittsburgh, Pa., June 16–19, 1991
Stereotact Funct Neurosurg 1992;58:59

Dorsal Selective Rhizotomy through a Limited Exposure of the Cauda Equina at L1

Giancarlo Barolat
Division of Functional Neurosurgery, Thomas Jefferson University, Philadelphia, Pa., USA

The technique of dorsal selective rhizotomy for the management of spasticity in cerebral palsy as originally developed by Prof. Fasano and by the author is described. The rhizotomy is performed through a one-level laminectomy at L1. Exposure of the conus medullaris and the cauda equina at this level is adequate to thoroughly assess the reflex electrical responses to stimulation of the lumbosacral roots and to perform the sectioning of the selected roots/rootlets. This approach, based on over 100 surgical procedures, obviates the need for an extensive laminectomy in a growing child without compromising the clinical results.

1011–6125/92/0584–0059 $ 2.75/0

Proceedings of the Meeting of the American Society for Stereotactic and Functional Neurosurgery, Pittsburgh, Pa., June 16–19, 1991
Stereotact Funct Neurosurg 1992;58:60–66

Pioneers of Stereotactic Neurosurgery

Nayef R.F. Al-Rodhan, Patrick J. Kelly

Department of Neurosurgery, Mayo Clinic and
Mayo Graduate School of Medicine, Rochester, Minn., USA

Key Words. Stereotactic neurosurgery · Neurosurgery history · Horsley · Medicine history · Surgical instruments

Abstract. The beginnings of stereotactic and functional neurosurgery can be traced as far back as 1873 when Dittmar reported the use of a guiding device for the placement of probes into the medulla oblongata in animals. Further pioneering work was done by Zernov and Altukhov in Russia (1889), Clarke and Horsley in England (1908), and Spiegel and Wycis in the United States (1947), as well as others. After a promising initiation, interest in stereotactic neurosurgery waned after the introduction of *L*-dopa in the 1960s. Later, the introduction and incorporation of new imaging technology into stereotactic techniques signaled the rebirth of stereotactic and functional neurosurgery as a versatile and exciting subspecialty not only in the resection of previously unresectable lesions but also in the functional restoration of central nervous system function. This brief paper will focus on the personalities that have pioneered stereotactic neurosurgery over the past century.

Introduction

Over the past century, stereotactic neurosurgery has developed from an investigational tool to study neuroscience to an exciting and significant part of modern neurosurgery. In this brief account, the personalities and their pioneering efforts in the development of stereotaxy will be discussed.

Leonardo da Vinci and René Descartes

The earliest sketch of a skull with three coordinate axes that could correspond to the same axes of the brain was drawn by Leonardo da Vinci in the late 15th century (fig. 1) [1]. Later it was possible to identify

1011–6125/92/0584–0060 $ 2.75/0

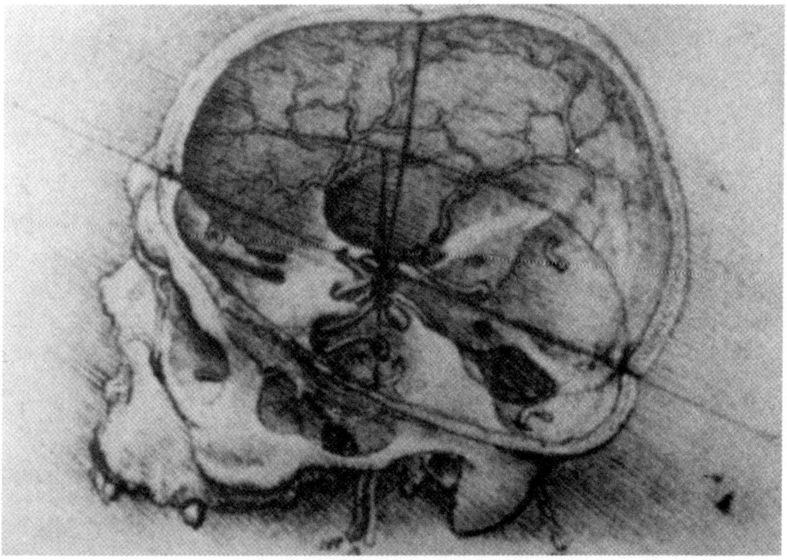

Fig. 1. The first sketch of three coordinate axes of the human skull by Leonardo da Vinci.

the position in space of a given structure using the cartesian system of rectangular, orthogonal coordinates, reciprocally perpendicular planes or polar coordinates. This was based on the work of the great French mathematician and philosopher René Descartes (1596–1650). The lines of intersection of the coordinate planes from three axes of the coordinate system, abscissa, ordina and applicata, all meet at one point referred to as the origin or zero point.

The Early Pioneers

The earliest documented use of the stereotactic principle in experimental work was by C. Dittmar who in 1873 [2] developed and used guiding devices for the placement of probes into the medulla oblongata of animals. These probes had three orthogonal degrees of precision although a coordinate system was not inherent in their usage. The next

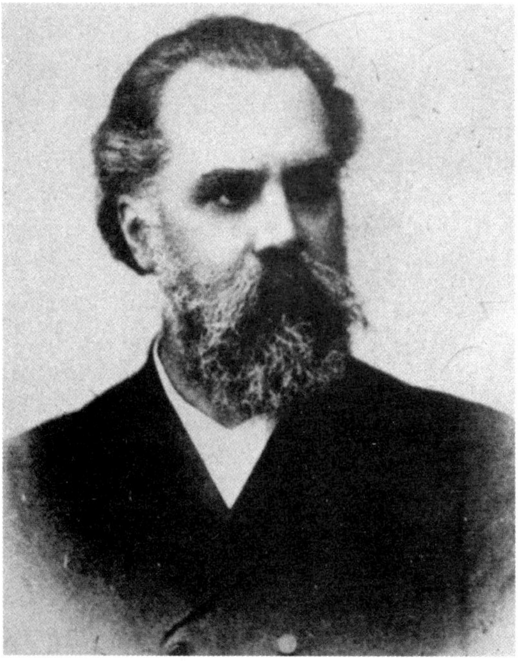

Fig. 2. Prof. D.N. Zernov of Moscow University (1876–1946).

development came from the laboratory of D.N. Zernov, Professor of Anatomy at Moscow University (fig. 2), who in 1889 [3] developed and reported a stereotactic apparatus called an encephalometer. This consisted of a basal ring, an equator and a meridian. It employed a system of polar coordinates for determining the position of deep as well as superficial structures. Its first human use was in 1889 when it was used to drain an intracranial abscess [4].

Horsley and Clarke

The efforts of these two men represent a milestone in neurosurgery. Sir Victor Horsley, a distinguished neurosurgeon and investiga-

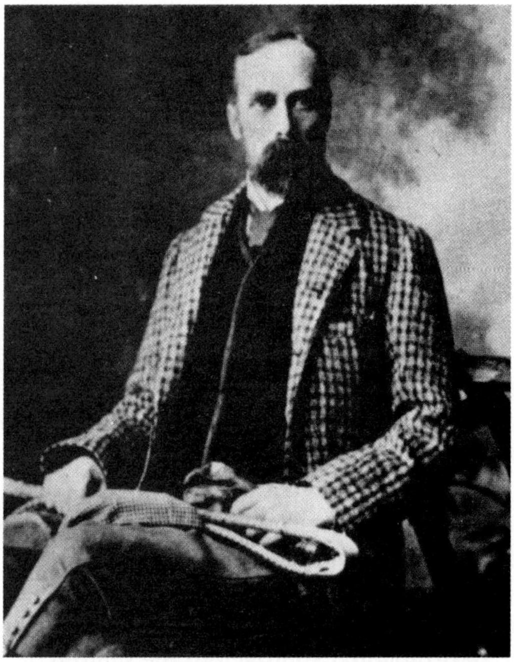

Fig. 3. Robert Henry Clarke of London (1850–1926).

tor, while studying the deep cerebellar nuclei wanted a reliable way to help insert an electrode in the dentate nucleus. In this effort, he was joined by Henry Clarke (fig. 3), another distinguished Victorian. The first of the Clarke instruments was made by James Swift in 1906 in London and followed by several other prototypes. Their work was published in 1906 and 1908 [5]. Their respective personalities led to the dissolution of their relationsship [6]. Horsley angered Clarke by discounting the possibility that this instrument could be used in humans, something that Clarke felt very strongly about. Clarke felt betrayed and his achievement belittled. On the other hand, Clarke was said to have been very bitter and jealous of Horsley's achievements as a famous scholar and as the King's surgeon. He accused him of being a self-seeking political wire-puller.

The Horsley-Clarke apparatus attached to the animal's skull by means of bars inserted into the external auditory canal and fixed to the hard palate and intraorbital ridge. The cranial fixation points established the baseline for a three-dimensional cartesian stereotactic coordinate system: the midline, the intraaxial plane and the canthomeatal plane.

The Early North American Stereotacticians

The introduction of the Horsley-Clarke device to the United States by Ernest Sachs of St. Louis in 1911 made a major impression on the early investigators interested in the field. This was started by Ranson and Hinsey in St. Louis in 1924 and later by Ranson and Ingram at Northwestern in 1932 and continued until Ranson's death in 1942.

The 'stereotactic' method also caught the interest of Aubrey Mussen who reproduced the Horsley-Clarke device that was purchased by the Johns Hopkins Hospital. Mussen built his own device for human use around 1918 which consisted of a rectangular brass frame with rectilinear coordinates for an orthogonal approach to the sagittal or coronal plane [7]. Unfortunately, Mussen was never able to convince a neurosurgeon to use his device.

The Rise and Decline of Stereotactic Neurosurgery

The increased interest in stereotaxy began with the German investigator Kirschner who in 1933 [8] described an instrument for the thermocoagulation of the gasserian ganglion. This consisted of a phantom measuring device on which the electrode laterality was set.

This was followed by the monumental work of Spiegel and Wycis in Philadelphia who were the second (after Zernov) to demonstrate that the stereotactic technique could be used in human neurosurgery. They designed several prototypes of stereotactic instruments and reported the first use in humans in North America in 1947 [9].

The important contributions of Spiegel and Wycis encouraged several investigators around the world to use the stereotactic technique experimentally as well as for human use. These included: Lars Leksell in Sweden; Umbach, Reichert and Mundinger in Germany;

Talairach, Szikla, Guit, Gros and Pecker in France; Narabayashi and Sano in Japan; Gillingham and Walsh in Britain; Obrador in Spain; Laitinen in Finland; Nadvornik in Czechoslavakia; Mempel in Poland; Kandel in the USSR; Meyers, Walker, Schaltenbrand, Cooper, Andy, Tasker, Nashold in the United States; Penfield, Bertrand and Hardy in Canada; Krayenbühl and Siegfried in Switzerland, and others.

This growth in the stereotactic method in the 1960s consisted mainly of neuroablative procedures for the treatment of movement disorders and chronic pain. Between 1960 and 1970, over 40,000 procedures were done with improved techniques and results. However, the introduction of *L*-dopa for Parkinson's disease in the late 1960s resulted in a rapid decline in interest and availability of stereotactic neurosurgery.

Modern Neurosurgery and the Future

The renaissance in stereotactic neurosurgery was primarily due to the incorporation of new imaging technologies into stereotactic techniques. The introduction of CT, MRI and improved computerized software revolutionized stereotactic neurosurgery. Because of the importance of technology in today's stereotactic neurosurgery, stereotactic neurosurgeons must keep themselves fully informed about emerging technologies in order to incorporate them into the stereotactic methodology.

The future of stereotactic neurosurgery is very bright and the possibilities are only limited by our imaginations.

References

1 Kandel EI: Functional and Stereotactic Neurosurgery. New York, Plenum, 1989.
2 Dittmar C: Über die Lage des sogenannten Gefässzentrums in der Medulla oblongata. Ber Sächs Ges Wiss, Leipzig (Math Phys) 1873;25:449–469.
3 Zernov DN: Encephalometer: Device for estimation of parts of brain in human (in Russian). Proc Soc Physicomed, Moscow 1889;2:70–80.
4 Altukhov NV: Encephalometric Investigations of the Brain Relative to the Sex, Age and Skull Indexes. Moscow, 1891.
5 Horsley V, Clarke RH: The structure and functions of the cerebellum examined by a new method. Brain 1908;31:45–124.

6 Davis RA: The surgeons's library. The book shelf. Victorian physician-scholar and pioneer physiologist. Surg Gynecol Obstet 1964;119:1333–1340.
7 Picard C, Olivier A, Bertrand G: The first human stereotaxic apparatus: The contribution of Aubrey Mussen to the field of stereotaxis. J Neurosurg 1983;59:673–676.
8 Kirschner M: Die Punktionstechnik und Elektrokoagulation des Ganglion Gasseri. Arch Klin Chir 1933;176:581–620.
9 Spiegel EA, Wycis HT, Marks M, et al: Stereotaxic apparatus for operations on the human brain. Science 1947;106:349–350.

Nayef Al-Rodhan, MD, Department of Neurosurgery, Mayo Clinic,
Rochester, MN 55905 (USA)

Proceedings of the Meeting of the American Society for Stereotactic and Functional Neurosurgery, Pittsburgh, Pa., June 16–19, 1991
Stereotact Funct Neurosurg 1992;58:67–78

Central Nervous System Grafting: Animal and Clinical Results

Roy A.E. Bakay

Department of Neurosurgery, Emory University School of Medicine, Atlanta, Ga., USA

Key Words. Parkinson's disease · Adrenal medulla · Co-graft · Fetal tissue · CNS graft

Abstract. In the 2 years since this topic was reviewed, there have been dramatic changes in our understanding of the basic science of central nervous system transplantation, as well as further realization of the crude state in which we find the clinical application of this technology. Early concepts of simple diffusion and neuronal replacement have been altered as we understand more the rule of neurotrophic factors and the response of the host to the transplantation process. Clinical studies are becoming increasingly sophisticated as we realize that the initial observations were frequently flawed and quantitative eveluations are increasingly important in determining the effectiveness of the procedure. There is, nervertheless, still a great deal of excitement in the field as new technologies are being developed and utilized in the clinical sphere.

Introduction

Parkinson's disease (PD) is a common degenerative disorder affecting over a half million people in the US. It produces progressive disability through dysfunction of the motor system. The major pathophysiological changes result from loss of dopaminergic neurons in the substantia nigra pars compacta. There are a number of exciting new therapeutic possibilities, including medication to slow down and retard the progression of the disease by presumably protecting the remaining dopaminergic neurons [1, 2]. New therapy also provides better medical management for those with symptoms of the disease by improving the consistency of dopamine release [3, 4]. Nevertheless, we have no cure.

1011–6125/92/0584–0067 $ 2.75/0

For patients with disability that is not adequately responsive to medication, the potential for therapy through ablative or reparative surgical intervention has been strengthened. Traditional ablative therapy has been most effective for tremor and rigidity, but has little effect in the most severely debilitating aspect of the disease, i.e. akinesia and bradykinesia. While thalamotomy remains effective for selected patients, a new understanding of the anatomy of the basal ganglia at a neurotransmitter level, combined with electrophysiological data from both normal and parkinsonian states, has led to consideration of new targets for ablative therapy [5]. Because akinesia and bradykinesia are the result of overactivity of the subthalamic nucleus and the globus pallidus pars interna, both nuclei have been suggested as targets for ablation. There is both old [6] and new [7] clinical data to suggest that these concepts are correct. In the past, pallidotomy lesioning was made in the wrong location. Currently, however, it is unclear whether these lesions are efficacious and safe enough to be used routinely.

The ultimate future treatment of many symptomatic neurological diseases rests with regenerative and reconstructive techniques. This technology will require an understanding of the basic pathophysiology of the neurological disease coupled with an understanding of the regenerative and/or restorative needs of the injured area. Reparative and regenerative therapy will for some time to come require the placement of central nervous system (CNS) grafts to provide functions that cannot be supplied by any other means. In pakinsonism, CNS grafting can be used to overcome dopamine deficiencies not only in neurotoxic models but also in genetic models of nigrostriatal degeneration [8, 9]. CNS grafts can be used to directly supply deficient neurotransmitters or neurotrophic factors, replace lost tissue, prevent loss of neural tissue, or provide a bridge to reestablish connection between two areas of the brain [10]. The potentials for therapeutic intervention using these techniques are extremely powerful.

What We Have Learned: Preclinical Studies

Grafting with fetal mesencephalic (FM) tissue has the theoretical advantage that the precise neurons required for reversal of the neurological deficit can be integrated into the host striatum. Grafted FM neurons in rats fire spontaneously and can be inhibited or activated by the host [11–13]. Grafted FM neurons have also demonstrated the ability to sustain intracranial self-stimulation, suggesting that under certain circumstances these grafted neurons axonally convey specific temporally organized information to the reinnervated striatum [14]. Behavioral recovery is related to the number of dopaminergic neurons in the graft [15], the extent of axonal reinnervation [16] and the topographic distribution [17]. Dopaminergic synaptic contacts from human FM grafts onto mouse hosts have been observed, and as the number of contacts increase there is a corresponding behavioral improvement [18]. Reports of FM grafts in monkeys have shown consistently improved behavior and survival of a significant number of neurons [19–25]. However, it is unclear whether anatomic integration of this degree is needed for optimal behavioral recovery, since recovery can be observed by FM grafts that may not reinnervate the host [24].

A major disadvantage of FM grafts is the difficulty in acquiring appropriate tissue, should this therapy ever be widely adopted for clinical treatment of PD. The legal and moral questions are complex. The use of cell culture lines and genetically engineered cells is very promising and may avoid the ethical issues [10], but it would not avoid the major disadvantage of any allograft technique, which is the risk of immunologic rejection and the potential initiation of an autoimmune encephalopathy. This risk appears small, but there are very few nonhuman primate studies upon which to draw inferences.

Grafting with adrenal medullary (AM) tissue has the advantage of utilizing autograft, with almost no risk of rejection or adverse immunologic reactions. Unfortunately, this tissue does not contain functional dopaminergic neurons. The chromaffin cells are capable of neuronal transformation in primates, but only under certain conditions [26–28]. Although biochemical differentiation to a state of increased dopamine synthesis and fiber formation can be seen in intracranial AM grafts, the chromaffin cells are rarely integrated into the host striatum and may simply serve as a 'catecholamine infusion pump'. There is disagreement whether it is dopamine [29] or a neurotrophic factor [30] that needs to be infused, or even if chromaffin tissue is required [31]. AM grafts do not appear to work as well as FM grafts in correcting turning behavior in the rat, especially in older animals [26]. Reports of AM grafts in monkeys demonstrate inconsistent behavioral improvement, probably due to poorer survival rate and much less neuronal differentiation compared to rats [32–38].

Because of the advantages of autografts, tissue of the sympathetic ganglia, retina and mesenteric ganglia should be further investigated as potential dopaminergic sources. Although tissues such as superior cervical ganglion are achieving modest success in human [39] and nonhuman [40] primate studies, the general consensus is that there are too few cells available and no substantial way to refine this technology to improve the results dramatically.

What We Have Learned: Clinical Studies

Despite this tremendous potential and almost 10-year history of application, CNS grafting has not played a significant clinical role. The first operation was performed in 1982 by Backlund using stereotactic techniques to implant AM tissue into the head of the right caudate nucleus. Two patients with advanced PD were studied and no significant improvement was observed [41]. Next, the number of implants was increased and a potentially superior target, the putamen, was used. Slightly better results were achieved in these younger and less severely involved patients. Nevertheless, the results were not felt to represent a significant degree of improvement [42]. It became obvious to the Swedish investigators that the AM tissue required nerve growth factor (NGF) for survival and conversion from an endocrine to a neuronal morphology. There is almost no NGF receptor or mRNA for NGF synthesis in the caudate of primates [43–45]. The original experiments were performed on rodents and grafted newborn AM tissue, which apparently has greater potential for survival than adult tissue [26]. NGF appeared to be essential even in rodent studies when adults were used as donors [46]. The next logical step was to graft AM tissue and infuse NGF to promote its survival and integration into the host. Preliminary results with this technique are promising, but the improvement still seems relatively small [47].

Against this background has been the very large worldwide attempt to reproduce the dramatic improvements reported by Madrazo et al. [48] by using a transcortical intraventricular craniotomy technique to place the AM tissue directly into the right caudate nucleus. There has been experimental evidence suggesting that the AM tissue is much more likely to survive in an intraventricular position than as an intraparenchymal graft [49]. However, the degree of improvement was considered to be mild to moderate, and the surgical morbidity and mortality was excessive [50, 51]. Nevertheless, a great deal of information was learned from these investigations. It is quite clear that some patients improved despite the small number of surviving AM cells in the graft, as suggested by autopsy data [52–58].

The induction of host regeneration is also a possible mechanism for recovery. Bohn et al. [30, 59] demonstrated that the grafting process itself may serve to induce 'sprouting' of the host residual dopaminergic cells. Studies from nonhuman primates seem to confirm this [35, 36]. We have demonstrated that the degree of improvement in our patients appears to correlate with the number of tyrosine-hydroxylase-immunoreactive (TH-ir) boutons present in the caudate at the time of grafting [60]. The amount of graft tissue and various demographic characteristics of the patient did not correlate with the recovery. This suggests that the greater the degree to which the host dopaminergic system has survived, the more likely the sprouting induced by release of neurotrophic factors will result in a clinically significant improvement. Most of the autopsy data from AM-grafted patients were not carefully analyzed. There are at least two autopsy reports suggesting that TH-ir fibers in the host are much more abundant around the graft site despite minimal TH-ir cell survival [57, 58]. The grafting process may have induced sprouting at least on a local level. The exact role of the grafted tissue remains to be determined.

The analysis of the clinical studies demonstrates less about what ensures a successful graft and more about what needs to be avoided. Aged and severely disabled patients are less likely to show clinically significant improvement predominantly because of the increased rate of complications that accompany age and disability [61]. However, an evaluation of the surgical technique revealed a statistically significant reduction in complications when the surgery was performed stereotactically [50]. This is a significant finding and one which must be incorporated in future clinical studies. We cannot change the patient's age and disability but we can alter our surgical techniques to provide a greater degree of safety. What remains to be determined is whether such techniques are equally efficacious. These are studies best suited for nonhuman primate investigation.

Stereotactic techniques also allow grafting into multiple sites. The principle for selecting multiple sites is founded in the rodent transplantation literature. Reinnervation of the rat striatum with FM grafts occurs over a very short distance and is never complete [16, 62]. It has been estimated that the maximum total reinnervation volume around a 1-mm graft is about 6 mm^3 [63]. Our experience with FM grafts in nonhuman primates suggests that the use of multiple injection sites leads to better results. Effects of AM grafting are also over a small area. Selection of the appropriate target sites is a critical variable to evaluate and control. The original rodent studies used an intraventricular placement of grafts or direct placement of FM grafts into the medial dorsal aspect of the striatum (the anatomic equivalent of the caudate). Carefully performed rodent studies demonstrated differences between ventral and dorsal placement of graft tissue [64] and the advisability of placing graft tissue in multiple locations to maximize improvement [16, 62]. Nonhuman primate AM grafting focused on the caudate almost exclusively [32–38]. Nonhuman primate studies using FM grafts have been more diverse in their choice of targets and most have used multiple targets in the host [19–25]. There has not been a systematic attempt in nonhuman primates to evaluate the caudate individually, the putamen individually, or both targets together. There are a number of reasons why the putamen may be an extremely important target. Previous grafting techniques have assumed that one area of putamen is of equal value to every other area. We now know the somatotropic distribution so that specific sites within the putamen can be targeted. Targeting of the putamen is not without risks. There are perforating arteries ascending from the ventral surface, which can produce a large area of infarction if damaged. It would be most useful to determine if grafting in this area is needed.

Only a few laboratories have investigated both FM and AM grafting techniques in nonhuman primates. Each of these investigators has indicated that FM appears superior to AM grafting [pers. communications]; however, none have studied these techniques concomitantly with statistical comparisons. Their evaluations also involved only AM grafting and not cografts. Chromaffin-Schwann cell cografts have been demonstrated unquestionably to provide superior graft survival [65, 66] and have demonstrated quantitative behavioral improvement [66]. A concomitant comparison using sufficient animals and quantitative behavioral techniques is therefore essential. A clinical study using cografts has been started.

Clinical investigations using FM tissue have yielded less dramatic results than had been anticipated. Part of the difficulties may relate to technical problems [67]. Recent review of the clinical FM grafting data, presented at the 1990 Fernstrom International Symposium in Lund, Sweden, suggested improvements which were of the same order of magnitude as many of the better AM grafting studies. The techniques used by various investigators demonstrate a tremendous diversity in approaches [10]. The number of fetuses per patient, the age of the fetal tissue, the preparation of the fetal tissue and the target selection are but a few of the differences among these studies. Any one of these variables could be critical to success. If these studies were large, altered some of the important variables and used randomized techniques, an answer to the best grafting technique might be anticipated. However, the number of patients is small and critical variables are not being randomized. Therefore, we must rely upon nonhuman primate studies to evaluate these important parameters. Many of these variables are being studied, but unfortunately not in a systematic manner and not with quantitative techniques. The technology is now available and an ever-increasing need to evaluate these techniques in nonhuman primates has resulted.

Conclusion

A number of questions regarding CNS transplantation simply cannot or should not be answered by clinical investigations. There is a tremendous need for data from controlled nonhuman primate studies to corroborate findings from clinical studies, to provide insight and rationales from the clinical observations, and to provide the basis for trying innovative techniques. The CNS transplantation for the treatment of PD is a reality. Laboratories worldwide are presently investigating CNS transplantation techniques for PD and other movement disorders. Current grafting technology needs refining in both the tissue and the surgical techniques. There is a need for multiple laboratory investigations of CNS grafting in nonhuman primates because of the number of variables involved and the diverse approaches used in both surgery and study design. The key factors to be identified in transplantation relate directly to donor tissue, implantation technique and recipient status. A number of host variables (age, severity of symptoms, duration of symptoms) are also important for successful transplantation. It is true that not all transplantation variables can be evaluated by laboratory studies.

Clinical trials are still essential. The models are not the disease and the ultimate test is the clinical trial. Clinical studies are needed to advance the laboratory finding, develop the techniques, and to generate problems for the laboratory. The clinical work adds relevance to the laboratory studies and stimulates activity. High-quality studies performed in both the laboratory and clinical setting are essential to provide the impetus for successful transplantation. The future is exciting.

References

1 Tetrud JW, Langston JW: The effects of deprenyl (selegiline) on the natural history of Parkinson's disease. Science 1989;245:519–522.
2 The Parkinson Study Group: The effects of deprenyl on the progression of disability in early Parkinson's disease. N Engl J Med 1989;321:1364–1371.
3 Koller WC, Hubble JP: Levodopa therapy in Parkinson's disease. Neurology 1990;40(suppl 3):40–47.
4 Goetz CG: Dopaminergic agonists in the treatment of Parkinson's disease. Neurology 1990;40(suppl 3):50–54.
5 Berman H, Wichmann T, DeLong MR: Reversal of experimental parkinsonism by lesions of the subthalamic nucleus. Science 1990;249:1436–1438.
6 Svennilson E, Torvik A, Lowe R, Leksell L: Treatment of parkinsonism by stereotactic thermolesions in the pallidal region. Acta Psychiatr Neurol Scand 1960; 35:358–377.
7 Laitinen LV, Bergenheim AT, Hariz MI: Leksell's posteroventral pallidotomy in the treatment of Parkinson's disease. J Neurosurg 1992;76:53–61.
8 Low WC, Triarhou LC, Kaseda Y, Norton J, Ghetti B: Functional innervation of the striatum by ventral mesencephalic grafts in mice with inherited nigrostriatal dopamine deficiency. Brain Res 1987;435:315–321.
9 Doucet G, Brundin P, Seth S, Murata Y, Strecker RE, Triarhou LC, Ghetti B, Bjorklund A: Degeneration and graft-induced restoration of dopamine innvervation in the weaver mouse neostriatum: A quantitative radioautographic study of [^{3}H]dopamine uptake. Exp Brain Res 1989;77:552–568.
10 Bakay RAE: Transplantation into the central nervous system: A therapy of the furture. Neurosurg Clin North Am 1990;1:881–895.
11 Wuerthele SM, Freed WJ, Olson L, Morihisa J, Spoor L, Wyatt RJ, Hoffer BJ: Effect of dopamine agonists and antagonists on the electrical activity of SN neurons transplanted into the lateral ventricle of the rat. Exp Brain Res 1981; 44:1–10.
12 Hoffer B, Rose G, Gerhardt G, Stromberg I, Olson L: Demonstration of monoamine release from transplant-reinnervated caudate nucleus by in vivo electrochemical detection; in Bjorklund A, Stenevi V (eds): Neural Grafting in the Mammalian CNS. Amsterdam, Elsevier, 1985, pp 437–447.
13 Bjorklund A, Lindvall O, Isacson O, Brundin P, Wictorin K, Strecker RE, Clarke

KJ, Dunnett SB: Mechanisms of action of interacerebral neural implants: Studies on nigral and striatal grafts to the lesioned striatum. Trends Neurosci 1987;10:509–516.

14 Fray PJ, Dunnett SB, Iversen SD, Bjorklund A, Stenevi U: SN transplants reinnervating the DA depleted neostriatum can sustain intracranial self-stimulation. Science 1982;219:416–419.

15 Brundin P, Isacson O, Bjorklund A: Monitoring of cell viability in suspension of embryonic CNS tissue and its use as a criterion for intracerebral grafts survival. Brain Res 1985;331:251–259.

16 Bjorklund A, Dunnett SB, Stenevi U, Lewis ME, Iverson SD: Reinnervation of the denervated striatum by substantia nigra transplants: Functional consequences as revealed by pharmacological and sensorimotor testing. Brain Res 1980;199:307–333.

17 Dunnett SB, Bjorklund A, Stenevi U, Iversen SD: Grafts of embryonic substantia nigra reinnervating the ventrolateral striatum ameliorate sensorimotor impairments and akinsesia in rats with 6-OHDA lesions of the nigrostriatal pathway. Brain Res 1981;229:209–217.

18 Clarke DJ, Brundin P, Strecker RE, Nilsson OG, Bjorklund A, Lindvall O: Human fetal dopamine neurons grafted in a rat model of Parkinson's disease: Ultrastructural evidence for synapse formation using tyrosine hydroxylase immunocytochemistry. Exp Brain Res 1988;73:115–126.

19 Bakay, RAE, Fiandaca MS, Barrow DL, Schiff A, Collins DC: Preliminary report on the use of fetal neural tissue transplantation to correct NMPTP induced primate model of parkinsonism. Appl Neurophysiol 1985;48:358–361.

20 Bakay RAE, Barrow DL, Fiandaca MS, Schiff A, Collins DC: Biochemical and behavioral correction of MPTP parkinson-like syndrome by fetal cell transplantation. Ann NY Acad Sci 1986;495:623–640.

21 Redmond DE Jr, Sladek JR Jr, Roth RH, Collier TJ, Elsworth JD, Deutch AY, Haber S: Fetal neuronal grafts in monkeys given methylphenyl tetrahydropyridine. Lancet 1986;i:1125–1127.

22 Dubach M, Schmidt RH, Martin R, German DC, Bowden DM: Transplants improves hemiparkinsonian syndrome in nonhuman primates: Intracerebral injection, rotometry, tyrosine hydroxylase immunohistochemistry. Prog Brain Res 1988;78:491–496.

23 Fine A, Hunt SP, Oertel WH, Nomoto M, Chong PN, Bond A, Water C, Temlett JA, Annett J, Dunnett S, Jenner PM, Marsden CD: Transplantation of embryonic marmoset dopaminergic neurons to the corpus striatum of marmosets rendered parkinsonian by MPTP. Prog Brain Res 1988;78:479–488.

24 Bankiewicz KS, Plunkett RJ, Jacobowitz DM: The effect of fetal mesencephalon implant on primate MPTP-induced parkinsonian: Histochemical and behavioral studies. Neurosurgery 1990;72:231–244.

25 Freed CR, Richards JB, Sabol KE, Reite ML: Fetal substantia nigra transplants lead to dopamine cell replacement and behavioral improvement in Bonnet monkeys with MPTP induced parkinsonism; in Beart PM, Woodruff G, Jackson DM (eds): Pharmacology and Functional Regulation of Dopaminergic Neurons. London, Macmillan, 1988, pp 353–360.

26 Freed WJ: Functional brain tissue transplantation: Reversal of lesion-induced ro-

tation by intraventricular SN and adrenal medulla grafts, with a note on intracranial retinal grafts. Biol Psychiatry 1983;18:1205–1266.

27 Patel-Vaidya U, Wells MR, Freed WJ: Survival of dissociated chromaffin cells of rat and monkey transplanted into rat brain. Cell Tissue Res 1984;240:281–285.

28 Lillien LE, Claude P: Nerve growth factor and glucocorticoids regulate phenotypic expression in cultured chromaffin cells from adult Rhesus monkeys. Exp Cell Res 1985;161:255–268.

29 Becker JB, Freed WJ: Neurochemical correlates of behavioral changes following intraventricular adrenal medulla grafts: Intraventricular microdialysis in freely moving rats. Prog Brain Res 1988;78:527–533.

30 Bohn MC, Marciano F, Cupit L, Gash DM: Recovery of dopaminergic fibers in striatum of the MPTP-treated mouse is enhanced by grafts of adrenal medulla. Prog Brain Res 1988;78:535–542.

31 Pezoli G, Fahn S, Dwork A, Truong DD, deYebenes JG, Jackson-Lewis V, Herbert J, Cadet JL: Non-chromaffin tissue + nerve growth factor reduces experimental parkinsonism in aged rats. Brain Res 1988;459:398–403.

32 Morihisa JM, Nakamura RK, Freed WJ, Mishkin M, Wyatt RJ: Adrenal medulla grafts survive and exhibit catecholamine-specific fluorescence in the primate brain. Exp Neurol 1984;84:643–653.

33 Watts RL, Bakay RAE: Autologous adrenal medulla-to-caudat grafting for parkinsonism in man and non-human primates. Frontiers of Endocrinology, in press.

34 Bakay RAE: What we have learned from primate research; in Lindvall O, Bjorklund A, Widner H (eds): Intracerebral Transplantation in Movement Disorders. Amsterdam, Elsevier, 1991, pp 53–66.

35 Fiandaca MS, Kordower JH, Hansen JT, Jiao SS, Gash DM: Adrenal medullary autografts into the basal ganglia of cebus monkeys: Injury-induced regeneration. Exp Neurol 1988;102:76–91.

36 Bankiewicz KS, Plunkett RJ, Kopin IJ, Jacobowitz DM, London WT, Oldfield EH: Transient behavioral recovery in hemiparkinsonian primates after adrenal medullary allografts. Prog Brain Res 1988;78:543–549.

37 Dubach M, German DC: Extensive survival of chromaffin cells in adrenal medullary 'ribbon' grafts in the monkey neostriatum. Exp Neurol 1990;110:167–180.

38 Yong VW, Guttman M, Kim SU, Calne DB, Turnbull I, Stabe K, Tomlinson RWW: Transplantation of human sympathetic neurons and adrenal chromaffin cells into parkinsonian monkeys: No reversal of clinical symptoms. Neuroscience 1989;94:51–67.

39 Horvath M, Pasztor E, Palikovits M, Solyom A, Tarczy M, Lekka N, Csanda E: Autotransplantation of superior cervical ganglion to the caudate nucleus in three patients with Parkinson's disease (preliminary report). Neurosurg Rev 1990;12: 119–122.

40 Itakura T, Kamei I, Nakai K, Naka Y, Nakakita K, Imai H, Komai N: Autotransplantation of the superior cervical ganglion into the brain: A possible therapy for Pakinson's disease. J Neurosurg 1988;68:955–959.

41 Backlund EO, Grandberg PO, Hamberger B, Knutso E, Martenson A, Sedball G, Seiger A, Olson L: Transplantation of adrenal medullary tissue to striatum in Parkinsonism: First clinical trials. J Neurosurg 1985;62:169–173.

bution, morphology, and colocalization with cholinergic enzymes. J Comp Neurol 1988;277:465–486.
42 Lindvall O, Backlund EO, Farde L: Transplantation in Parkinson's disease: Two cases of adrenal medullary grafts to the putamen. Ann Neurol 1987;22:457–468.
43 Kordower JH, Bartus RT, Bothwell M, Schattman G, Gash DM: Nerve growth factor receptor immunoreactivity in the nonhuman primate *(Cebus apella):* Distri-
44 Hayashi M, Yamashita A, Shimizu K: Nerve growth factor in the primate central nervous system: Regional distribution and ontogeny. Neuroscience 1990;36:683–689.
45 Schatteman GC, Gibbs L, Lanahan A, Claude P, Bothwell M: Expression of NGF receptor in the developing and adult primate central nervous system. J Neurosci 1988;8:860–873.
46 Stromberg I, Herrera-Marschitz M, Ungerstedt U, Edendal T, Olson L: Chronic implants of chromaffin tissue into the dopamine-denervated striatum: Effects of NGF on graft survival, fiber growth and rotational behavior. Exp Brain Res 1985;60:335–349.
47 Olson L, Backlund E-O, Ebendal T, Freedman R: Intraputaminal infusion of nerve growth factor to support adrenal medullary autografts in Parkinson's disease. Arch Neurol 1991;48:373–381.
48 Madrazo I, Drucker-Colin R, Diaz V, Martinez-Mata J, Torres C, Becerril JJ: Open microsurgical autograft of adrenal medulla to the right caudate nucleus in two patients with Parkinson's disease. N Engl J Med 1987;316:831–834.
49 Freed WJ, Cannon-Spoor HE, Krauthamer E: Intrastriatal adrenal medulla in rats. J Neurosurg 1986;65:664–670.
50 Bakay, RAE, Allen GS, Apuzzo M, Penn R, Tindall GT: Preliminary report on adrenal medullary grafting from the American Association of Neurological Surgeons, GRAFT project: Preliminary report. Prog Brain Res 1990;82:603–610.
51 Goetz CG, Stebbins GT III, Klawans HL, Koller WC, Grossman RG, Bakay RAE, Penn RD: United Parkinson Foundation Neurotransplantation Registry: Multicenter US and Canadian data base, presurgical and 12 month follow-up. Prog Brain Res 1990;82:611–617.
52 Dohan FC, Robertson JT, Feler C, Schweitzer J, Hall C, Robertson JH: Autopsy findings in a Parkinson's disease patint treated with adrenal medullary to caudate nucleus transplant. Soc Neurosci Abstr 1988;7:4.
53 Jankovic J, Grossman R, Goodman C: Clinical, biochemical, and neuropathologic findings following transplantation of adrenal medulla to the caudate nucleus for treatment of Parkinson's disease. Neurology 1989;39:1227–1234.
54 Hurtig HI, Trojanowski JQ, Joyce J, Sladek JR Jr, Goldstein M: Post mortem analysis of adrenal-medulla-to-caudate autograft in a patient with Parkinson's disease. Ann Neurol 1989,25:607–614.
55 Waters C, Itabashi HH, Apuzzo JLJ, Weiner LP: Adrenal to caudate transplantation: Postmortem study. Mov Disord 1990;5:248–250.
56 Peterson DI, Price ML, Small CS: Autopsy findings in a patient who had an adrenal-to-brain transplant for Parkinson's disease. Neurology 1989;39:235–238.
57 Hirsh EC, Duyckaerts C, Javoy-Agid F, Hauw JJ, Agid Y: Does adrenal graft enhance recovery of dopamine neurons in Parkinson's disease. Ann Neurol 1990;27:676–682.

58 Kordower JH, Cochran E, Penn RD, Goetz CG: Clinical assessment and neuropathological evaluation of a patient with Parkinson's disease surviving thirty months following an adrenal chromaffin cell autograft. Ann Neurol 1991;29:405–412.

59 Bohn MC, Cupit F, Marciano F, Gash DM: Adrenal medulla grafts enhance recovery of striatal dopaminergic fibers. Science 1987;237:913–916.

60 Bakay RAE, Watts RL, Freeman A, Iuvone PM, Watts NB, Graham SD: Preliminary report on adrenal-brain transplantation for parkinsonism in man. Stereotact Funct Neurosurg 1990;54/55:312–323.

61 Bakay RAE: Selection criteria for CNS grafting into Parkinson's disease patients; in Lindvall O, Oetal H (eds): Intracerebral Transplantation in Movement Disorders. Amsterdam, Elsevier, 1991, pp 137–148.

62 Dunnett SB, Bjorklund A, Gage FH, Stenevi U: Transplantation of mesencephalic dopamine neurons to the striatum of adult rats; in Bjorklund A, Stenevi U (eds): Neural Grafting in the Mammalian CNS. Amsterdam, Elsevier, 1985, pp 451–469.

63 Freed WJ, Cannon-Spoor HE, Drauthamer E: Factors influencing the efficacy of adrenal medulla and embryonic SN grafts; in Bjorklund A, Stenevi U (ed): Neural Grafting in the Mammalian CNS. Amsterdam, Elsevier, 1985, pp 491–504.

64 Dunnett SB, Bjorklund A, Schmidt RH, Stenevi U, Iversen SD: Intracerebral grafting of neuronal cell-suspensions. IV. Behavioral recovery in rats with bilateral 6-OHDA lesions following implantation of nigral cell suspensions. Acta Physiol Scand Suppl 1983;522:229–237.

65 Kordower JH, Fiandaca MS, Notter MFD, Hansen JT, Gash DM: NGF-like trophic support from peripheral nerve for grafted rhesus adrenal chromaffin cells. J Neurosurg 1990;73:418–428.

66 Watts RL, Bakay RAE, Herring CJ, et al: Preliminary report on adrenal medullary grafting and cografting with sural nerve in the treatment of hemiparkinson monkeys. Prog Brain Res 1990;82:581–591.

67 Lindvall O, Brundin P, Widner H, et al: Grafts of fetal dopamine neurons survive and improve motor function of Parkinson's disease. Science 1990;247:574.

Roy A.E. Bakay, MD, Department of Neurosurgery,
Emory University School of Medicine, 1327 Clifton Road, N.E.,
Atlanta, GA 30322 (USA)

Proceedings of the Meeting of the American Society for Stereotactic and Functional Neurosurgery, Pittsburgh, Pa., June 16–19, 1991
Stereotact Funct Neurosurg 1992;58:79–83

Stereotactic Technique and Pathophysiological Mechanisms of Neurotransplantation in Huntington's Chorea

M. Šramka[a], M. Rattaj[a], H. Molina[b], J. Vojtaššák[c], V. Belan[a], E. Ružický[a]

[a] Department of Stereotactic and Functional Neurosurgery, Institute of Preventive and Clinical Medicine, Bratislava, CSFR; [b] Iberolatinoamerican Center for Transplantation and Regeneration of Nervous System, Habana, Cuba

Key Words. Neurotransplantation · Huntington's chorea · Stereotaxy method · Embryonal brain tissue · Striatum

Abstract. In Huntington's chorea, embryonal brain tissue (striatum) was implanted in the caudate nucleus bilaterally, using stereotaxy assisted by CT. A special cannula allowed the placement into the brain of 3 or 4 grafts of embryonal tissue along the determined trajectory by one introduction of the cannula. The pathophysiological mechanism of neurotransplantation in Huntington's chorea is to compensate for the degenerated striatal tissue by embryonal striatum, so it is necessary to supply a quantity of embryonal striatal tissue which enables the whole functional integrity. Therefore, we use material from several embryos.

Experiments in animal models show that transplantation of brain tissue enables the regeneration of morphological connecting and biochemical functions [1]. Suitable anatomic placement for transplantation and also the conditions of survival have been determined. Madrazo et al. [2] from Mexico transplanted embryonal brain tissue from the substantia nigra area in the mesencephalon into the caudate nucleus of parkinsonian patients. Later, embryonal tissue of the mesencephalon was transplanted stereotactically [3].

In our department, stereotactic transplantation of embryonal mesencaphalic tissue into parkinsonian patients was performed in 1989 [4]. Transplantation of embryonal brain tissue into the striatum in Huntington's chorea was performed via open neurosurgery in Cuba and stereotactically in Czechoslovakia in 1990 [5].

1011–6125/92/0584–0079 $ 2.75/0

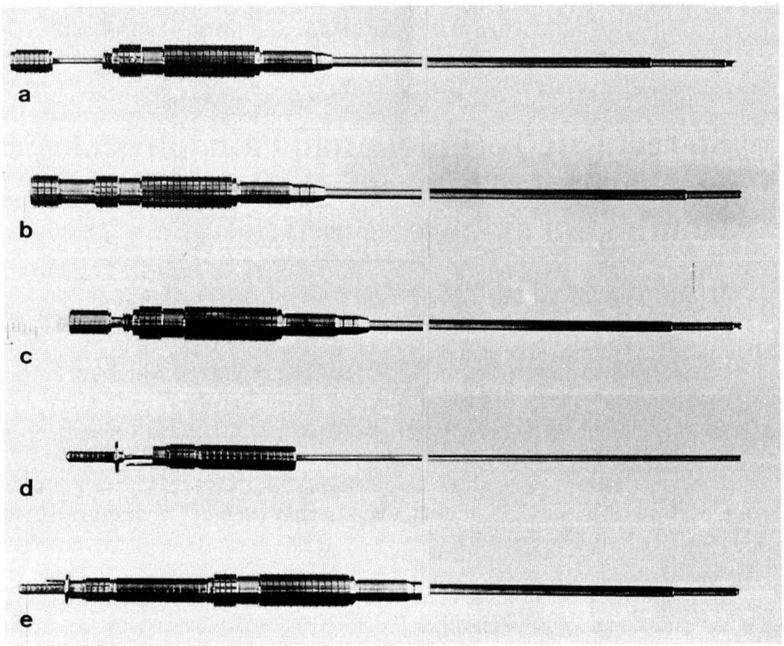

Fig. 1. Cannulas for neurotransplantation in Huntington's chorea. **a** Cannula with sharp mandrel. **b** Cannula with blunt mandrel. **c** Biopsy cannula. **d** Cannula with Teflon mandrel. **e** Double cannula for pick-up method. The cannulas for neurotransplantation were constructed by Mr. Gustav Mates in the Institute of Measurement Techniques, Slovak Academy of Science, Bratislava, CSFR.

Material and Technique

Embryonal tissue is obtained by extraction and vacuum aspiration under ultrasonic control. It is kept in Ringer's lactate solution at 4 °C under aseptic conditions and must be transplanted within 1 h after withdrawal. Before surgery, experimental verification of embryonal tissue is done.

For transplantation of embryonal tissue it is necessary to specify the physiological condition and the period of survival of the transplanted tissue. NMR spectroscopy is a noninvasive method which does not influence the metabolism of cells during the measurement, as can be verified by the fact that ATP concentration is nearly constant during the 2-hour storage.

Our transplantation technique consists of stereotaxy controlled by CT. The Reichert-Mündiger stereotactic apparatus is used. A special cannula of our own construction (fig. 1) enables us to place into the brain 3 or 4 tissue samples on the determined trajec-

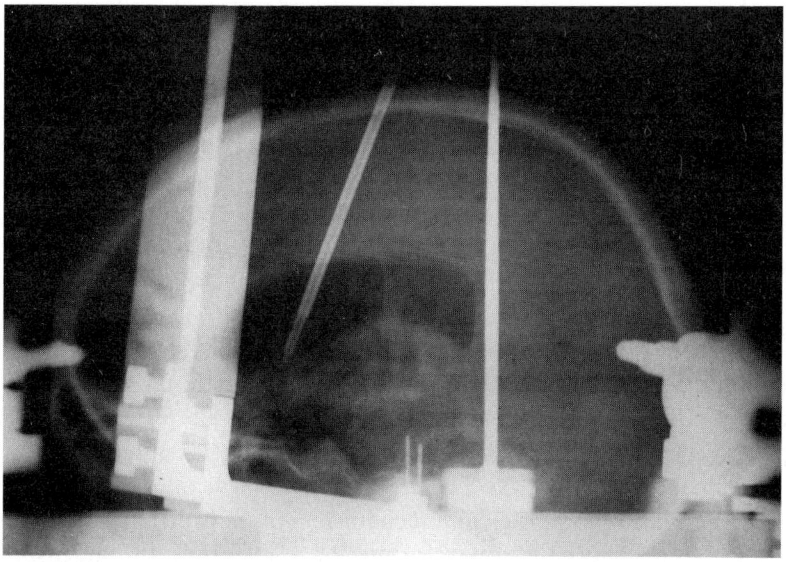

Fig. 2. Stereotactic neurotransplantation in Huntington's chorea. Biopsy cannula in the caput nuclei caudati (X-ray, lateral view).

tory by one introduction of the cannula without repetition. The set includes a biopsy cannula for the withdrawal of brain tissue of different shapes (for biochemical and histological examinations). The prepared 0.5-mm-thick strips of embryonal mesencephalon are placed into the cannula and implanted into the bed of the caput nuclei caudati (fig. 2), symmetrically on both sides. We used 2 or 3 embryos in every case. Embryonal tissue was successively applied into 4 or 5 loci of both caudate nuclei.

Results

The pre- and postoperative status is evaluated in a standard way by a scale used for Huntington's chorea. In operated patients we did not observe any pathological immunologic response, under the shielding of cyclosporin. The level of cyclosporin ranged from 150 to 250 mg/ml and was regularly examined. We did not observe any disturbance of kidney function in our patients.

Four patients with Huntington's chorea were transplanted with embryonal brain tissue. Intensive choreoathetosis with serious damage of the postural musculature and dystonia developed in these patients, mainly on voluntary movement, as well as in the lying position. They were in groups IV–V of the Hoehn-Yahr scale, and were not able to stand and walk. As yet it is not possible to make a final postoperative evaluation, but a reduction in amplitude and frequency of hyperkinesia has been observed.

Discussion

Recent experimental studies [6, 7] showed that striatal tissue grafted into denervated neostriatum promotes functional recovery. This model may prove the presumption that graft tissue provides at least a partial reconstruction of both the afferent and efferent components of the damaged circuits [8].

The pathophysiological mechanisms of neurotransplantation in Huntington's chorea and parkinsonism are different. In parkinsonism, the tissue of the substantia nigra producing a neurotransmitter is damaged, and embryonal mesencephalon is implanted directly into the normal striatum, so the graft can produce missing neurotransmitter, theoretically. Mostly, it is sufficient to implant the graft on one side only, because the small quantity of the graft saturates the insufficiency of neurotransmitter. In Huntington's chorea we compensate the degenerated striatal tissue by embryonal striatum. This suggests a different approach to neurotransplantation in parkinsonism and Huntington's chorea. It is necessary to compensate for the degenerated striatum in patients with Huntington's chorea and to supply a sufficient quantity of embryonal striatal tissue to enable the whole integrity of function. Therefore, we use material from usually 2–3 embryos. It is hoped to introduce tissue cultures of embryonal striatum into clinical practice [9].

References

1 Björklund A, Dunnett SB, Stenevi U, Lewis ME, Iversen SD: Reinnervation of the denervated striatum by substantia nigra transplants: Functional consequences as revealed by pharmacological and sensorimotor testing. Brain Res 1980;199:307–333.

2 Madrazo I, Leon V, Torres C, Del Carmen Aguilera M, Varela G, Alvarez F, Fraga A, Drucker-Colin R, Ostrovsky F, Skurovich M, Franco R: Transplantation of

fetal substantia nigra and adrenal medulla to the caudate nucleus in two patients with Parkinsons disease. N Engl J Med 1988;318:51.
3 Hitchcock ER, Kenny BG, Ciough CG, Hughes RC, Henderson BTH, Betta A: Stereotactic implantation of fetal mesencephalon (STIM). Abstr X Meet World Soc for Stereotactic and Functional Neurosurgery, Maebashi, Oct 1989, p 25.
4 Šramka M, Rattaj M, Vojtaššák J, Rusňák I, Belan V,Ružický E: Transplantation of embryonal tissue in treatment of Parkinson disease and Huntington's chorea. Int Congr of Bioenergetical and Biological Medicine. SSPKN, Bratislava, 1990, pp 39–40.
5 Molina H, Šramka M, Alvarez L, Vojtaššák J, Naranjo R, Rattaj M, Quinónez R, Rattaj J, Santana A, Rusnák I, Cordova F: Neurotransplantation in Huntington's chorea. Abstr 9th Congr Eur Soc for Stereotactic and Functional Neurosurgery, Marbella, Sept 1990, pp 54–56.
6 Deckel AW, Robinson RG, Coyle JT, Sanberg PR: Reversal of long-term locomotor abnormalities in the kainic acid model of Huntington's disease by day 18 fetal striatal implants. Eur J Pharmacol 1983;93:287–288.
7 Björklund A, Lindvall O, Isacson O, Brundin P, Wictorin K, Strecker RE, Clarke DJ, Dunnett SB: Mechanisms of action of intracerebral neural implants. Trends Neurosci 1987;10:509–516.
8 Dunnett SB, Isacson O, Sirinathsinghyi DJS, Clarke DJ, Björklund A: Striatal grafts in rats with unilateral neostriatal lesions. III. Recovery from dopamine dependent motor asymmetry and deficits in skilled paw reaching. Neuroscience 1988;24:813–820.
9 Ren Ben, Fan Ji-Chang, Bao Yao-Dong, Liu Yie-Jian, Zhang Yi-Fang: Transplantation of foetal adrenal medullary tissue culture to the head of caudate nucleus in 17 Parkinsonians. Abstr 9th Congr Eur Soc for Stereotactic and Functional Neurosurgery. Marbella, Sept 1990, pp 50–52.

M. Šramka, Department of Stereotactic and Functional Neurosurgery,
Derer's Hospital, Limbova str. 5, Bratislava (CSFR)

Proceedings of the Meeting of the American Society for Stereotactic and Functional Neurosurgery, Pittsburgh, Pa., June 16–19, 1991
Stereotact Funct Neurosurg 1992;58:84–87

Bilateral Fetal Grafts for Parkinson's Disease: 22 Months' Results

R.P. Iacono[a], *Z.S. Tang*[a], *J.C. Mazziotta*[b], *S. Grafton*[b], *M. Hoehn*[c]

[a] Department of Neurosurgery, Hua Shan Hospital, Shanghai, ROC;
[b] Department of Neurology and Radiology, UCLA School of Medicine, Calif., USA;
[c] Neurology, Denver, Colo., USA

Key Words. Fetal brain graft · Stereotactic surgery · Parkinson's disease

Abstract. Five patients with severe Parkinson's disease underwent bilateral multiple graft implants of nondissociated fetal mesodiencephalic tissues. Graft implantation was performed in China following CT-guided stereotactic placement of a novel delivery system. Follow-up has demonstrated substantially reduced levodopa requirements and clinical improvements of motor, postural functions and reduction of freezing and on-off phenomenon. PET utilizing [^{18}F]-dopa, at 14 months in the first case, suggested graft-induced restoration of dopaminergic transmission in the striatum.

The ability of fetal mesencephalic grafts to survive and result in symptomatic improvements in patients with Parkinson's disease (PD) has been documented [1]. This report discusses such grafting utilizing a different technique, and demonstrates that a therapeutically and socially valuable recovery can occur.

Methods

Five patients with Hoehn and Yahr grade III–IV PD underwent bilateral grafting of fetal mesodiencephalic tissues using nondissociated tissue fragments placed into the caudate and putamen nuclei bilaterally through stereotactically preimplanted specially designed polyethylene devices (AD-TECH; Racine, Wisc., USA). Using Brown-Roberts-Wells and Kumai CT-guided stereotactics, these catheters were placed into the caudate and putamen nuclei bilaterally, implanted through a twist-drill hole and the

1011–6125/92/0584–0084 $ 2.75/0

scalp was closed over them. Two to 11 days later the catheters were employed for sequential tissue implants carried out over a 2- to 4-day period [2]. In each patient, tissue samples were obtained from 2 or 3 newly aborted fetuses following guidelines set down by the NIH ethics committee; tissue implantation was carried out in China. Tissue was dissected into 0.5- to 1.5-mm pieces and either injected in a small volume as a suspension or loaded into an Apuzzo insertion coil and implanted [3]. The catheters were immediately removed over an obturator placed to ensure target depth positioning of the coils A tissue suspension was also injected into the ventricular system via an Ommaya reservoir [4, 5]. The volume of each implant was approximately 25 mm^3, or a total of 125 mm^3. Time from tissue access to implantation was 30–60 min. All implant procedures were performed with local anesthesia and required no additional CT, stereotactic or X-ray control. Patients received ciclosporin and prednisone immuno-suppression, beginning 48 h before, grafting with 10 mg/kg/day and 60 mg/day, respectively.

Results

Patient follow-up now ranges from 2 to 22 months, and has demonstrated substantially reduced (25–50%) levodopa requirements and clinical improvements of motor, postural and other functions, including reduction of freezing and on-off phenomenon, resolution of micrographia and hypophonia.

The first patient's clinical course was initially marked by the development of dilated pupils and enhanced sympathotonia, beginning 72 h following the completion of grafting and clearing over 6 h [6]. Thereafter, for approximately 6 weeks the patient's clinical condition was somewhat worse due to an enforced 50% reduction in his *L*-dopa medications. During this time (and as preoperatively) he required nursing care. The patient was admitted to the hospital every 4–6 weeks for intense observation. Videotape assessment was conducted at 3-month intervals. The patient showed improvements in facial expression at 6 weeks, followed shortly by improvement in speech, swallowing and in the quality of gait during on time. At 3.5 months, propulsions and postural instability improved. At 5.5 months the patient showed improvement in on-off. Freezing spells resolved. Between 6 months and 1 year there was a noticeable improvement in the smoothness of his gait. He was no longer dependent on a single dose of medication. At 15 months, specific as well as overall improvements on the Unified PD Rating Scales were noted (M.H.), compared with examination 3 years before surgery. At this time he could go 8 h on a single dose of levodopa. Neuropsychological evaluation revealed improvements in some aspects of cognitive functions, including reversal of sensory neglect over the previous year's evaluations. This patient whose severe pregraft PD was rated as Hoehn and Yahr stage IV–V, was rated by independent neurologists' examination as stage II–III, and he was able to resume full independent daily activities. However, he died suddenly 23 months following implantation; preliminary pathological findings are pending.

The surviving 4 patients, now 2–6 months after operation, have experienced similar improvements to date, and are demonstrating a very similar sequence of recovery of neurological function as the first patient, related to improvements of akinesia. No infections or immunosuppression-related problems have occurred.

PET was performed utilizing [18F]-labeled *L*-dopa (FD) 15 months (patient 1) and 6 months (patient 2) postoperatively at UCLA. The FD images were compared to those previously obtained in normal volunteers and patients with PD. Different from other patients with PD (patient 1) was an area of uptake slightly lateral and posterior to the left caudate nucleus. In addition, there was uptake in the posterior portion of the left putamen and on the left side of the pons. There was no specific uptake of FD in the ventricles.

Discussion

The preparation of a patient with PD for delayed multiple fetal brain grafts using an alternative stereotactic implant technique is described. This method minimizes time from tissue availability to implantation and allows sequential use of multiple tissue samples without repeat stereotactic procedures, simplifying the graft implantation procedues which involved the use of fresh tissue samples in sequence. Interpretation that the reduction in symptoms in these patients is due to neurochemical changes, including dopaminergic reinnervation of the striatum by the surviving and functioning graft, is supported by the PET findings of increased presynaptic uptake in the region of the grafted striata 14 months after the surgery, the progressive neurological improvements consistent with that of graft-induced changes in the studies, and long-term benefit. However, nongraft of nondopaminergic mechanisms may be important for the symptomatic improvements [7–9]. Caution as well as openmindedness are indicated in our further clinical investigations.

References

1 Lindvall O, Brudin P, Winoner H: Grafts of fetal dopamine neurons survive and improve motor functions in Parkinson's disease. Science 1990;247:574–577.
2 Bakay RAE, Fiandaca MS, Sweeney KM, Colbassari HJ: Delayed stereotactic transplantation technique in non-human primates. Prog Brain Res 1988;78:463–477.
3 Apuzzo MLJ, Neal JH, Waters CH: Utilization of unilateral and bilateral stereotactically placed adrenomedullary-striatal autografts in Parkinsonian humans: Rational, techniques and obsevations. Neurosurgery 1990;26:746–757.
4 Freed WJ, Dyneck J, Poltorak M: Intraventricular brain allografts and xenografts: Studies of survival and rejection with and without systemic sensitization. Brain Res 1988;78(chapt 30).
5 Nishino H, Ono T, Takahashi J, Rimura M, Saioaka S: Transplants in the peri- and intraventricular region grow better than those in the central parenchyma of the caudate. Neurosci Lett 1986;64:184–190.
6 Iacono RP, Van Dalen JTW: Transient pupillary abnormalities following fetal brain transplantation for Parkinson's disease. Neuro-Ophthal 1989;9:355–356.
7 Sandyk R, Iacono RP, Bamford C: The hypothalamus in Parkinson's disease. Ital J Neurol Sci 1987;8:227–234.
8 Bankiewica KS, Plunket RJ, Jacobowitz DM, Kopin IJ, Oldifield EH: Fetal non-dopaminergic implants in parkinsonian primates. J Neurosurg 1991;74:97–104.
9 Iacono RP, Sandyk R: Non-dopaminergic mechanisms in adrenal medullary transplantation for Parkinson's disease. Int J Neurosci 1989;45:259–260.

R.P. Iacono, 93 Saddleback Road, Rolling Hills, CA 90274 (USA)

Proceedings of the Meeting of the American Society for Stereotactic and Functional Neurosurgery, Pittsburgh, Pa., June 16–19, 1991
Stereotact Funct Neurosurg 1992;58:88

MR-Guided Ventral Intermediate Thalomotomy for Posttraumatic Hemiballismus

M.F. Levesque, C. Markham, N. Nakasato
Department of Neurosurgery, UCLA Medical Center, Los Angeles, Calif., USA

Hemiballismus is a rare type of dystonia and is usually caused by a vascular lesion involving the subthalamic nucleus. We are reporting the case of a 37-year old left-handed male who presented with medically intractable left hemiballismus of 21 years duration. After a closed head injury at age 16, he remained comatose for 3 weeks and underwent extensive rehabilitation for the following year. Neurologically, he was left with a mild dysarthria and a constant flinging movement of the left upper extremity, involving mainly the proximal arm and shoulder musculature, with slight increase in tone but no motor deficit. There was no associated torticollis, palatal myoclonus or family history of dystonia. Neuroimaging studies were entirely normal. A stereotactic MR-guided ventral intermediate thalamotomy was performed on the right side under local anesthesia with an immediate improvement in the constant hemiballismus. In the following 2 days, there was a complete resolution of the dystonia which persisted after 9 months of follow-up. Postoperatively, a mild cerebellar ataxia and a moderate dysarthria were neurologically present. Postoperative MR studies disclosed the accuracy and size of the lesion.

1011–6125/92/0584–0088 $ 2.75/0

Proceedings of the Meeting of the American Society for Stereotactic and Functional Neurosurgery, Pittsburgh, Pa., June 16–19, 1991
Stereotact Funct Neurosurg 1992;58:89

Excision of Arteriovenous Malformation in Sensorimotor and Language-Related Neocortex Using Stimulation Mapping and Corticography under Local Anesthesia

John P. Gorecki, Robert R. Smith, Abelardo S. Wee
Department of Neurosurgery, University of Mississippi Medical Center, Jackson, MS, USA

Arteriovenous malformations (AVMs) are dealt with using a variety of techniques including direct excision (attacking arterial feeders or by retrograde isolation), controlled hypotension, endovascular intervention, stereotactic irradiation, staged operations and direct cortical mapping. Rolandic AVMs are particularly challenging. Compromise of vascular supply to normal surrounding brain or direct trauma to eloquent neocortex may result in unacceptable neurological morbidity. In patients with epilepsy, failure to excise areas of epileptogenic brain as identified by corticography may result in continued seizures, after successful obliteration of the AVM. In this report, we describe 2 patients who underwent excision of large rolandic AVMs under local anesthesia. One lesion was located in the dominant (left) hemisphere. Both patients underwent pre- and postoperative neuropsychological evaluation. The WADA test was not performed since there was no language ambiguity. Electrocorticography was used to identifiy epileptogenic brain. Stimulation-mapping techniques were used to identify critical motor, sensory and language areas. The resection was carried out at the same procedure allowing ongoing testing of neurological function as feeding vessels were taken. Both patients demonstrated delayed, transient deficits as anticipated which resolved over 7–14 days. Cortical mapping under local anesthesia is beneficial for resection of certain AVMs located in eloquent areas and it is not necessary to perform a second operation under general anesthesia to excise the lesions.

1011–6125/92/0584–0089 $ 2.75/0

Proceedings of the Meeting of the American Society for Stereotactic and Functional Neurosurgery, Pittsburgh, Pa., June 16–19, 1991
Stereotact Funct Neurosurg 1992;58:90–93

Computer and Imaging Technology's Impact on Stereotactic Neurosurgery

A 1987–1991 Update

Bruce A. Kall

Mayo Clinic, Section of Patient Care Systems, Rochester, Minn., USA

Key Words. Computers · Imaging · Stereotactic treatment planning

Abstract. Many improvements in computer and imaging technology have occurred since the last meeting of the American Society for Stereotactic and Functional Neurosurgery in 1987. These improvements are leading to a much wider acceptance of computerization and computer-assisted surgical procedures in the stereotactic neurosurgery field. This paper surveys the current fields of computer and imaging technology and its relationship and impact on the field of stereotactic neurosurgery during the period of 1987–1991. Forecasts about future developments are also discussed.

Introduction

Computers and imaging technology continue to have a significant impact on stereotactic neurosurgery. Continually improving computing has led to less expensive yet significantly faster and capacious computers. Imaging technology, and more specifically radiological scanning, is improving as a result of further research and development, but it too, is impacted by the evolution of faster computers resulting in a new generation of scanners. Advances in visualization and quantitative analysis of imaging data as well as further refinement in stereotactic software will continue to advance the diagnostic and therapeutic qualities of stereotactic treatment-planning systems.

This paper will review some of the more important developments that have occurred since the last meeting of the American Society of Stereotactic and Functional Neurosurgery (ASSFN) in Montreal in

1011–6125/92/0584–0090 $ 2.75/0

June 1987. An outlook for the future 1990s technological innovations that may impact stereotactic neurosurgery will also be discussed.

The Years 1987–1991

Many significant new developments have occurred since the last meeting of ASSFN in 1987. Integration of MRI into stereotaxis was well underway in 1987. Today, *magnetic resonance angiography* promises to be a noninvasive means for localizing the vascular structures for stereotactic procedures. Integration, comparison and fusing of multimodality radiological images was also a topic during the 1987 meeting. Integration of voice, sound, image and text is a currently the subject of much research and development and is called *multimedia.*

Workstations, usually composed of high-powered UNIX-based computers with high-resolution graphics screens, are beginning to overtake personal computers in the number of applications available for stereotactic neurosurgery. Workstation performance, as measured in million instructions per second (MIPS), has roughly doubled each year since 1987. The Sun Microsystems 3/260 was a leader in workstation technology at 4 MIPS in 1987. Currently, the Hewlett-Packard model 750 is rated at 76 MIPS.

An operating system is a combination of a command language and a variety of utility programs that are utilized to control the basic functions and manage the resource of a computer. IBM's OS/2 was heralded as the operating system of the future for personal computers in 1987. *Microsoft Windows,* sitting on top of older technology DOS, has already overtaken OS/2 in 1991 as the graphic operating system of choice for IBM and compatible computers. *UNIX,* an operating system developed by AT&T many years ago, is already the operating system of choice on workstations and will be adopted on more and more next-generation personal computers.

Networking technology has also undergone advancements since 1987 when modems and Ethernet were the methods of interconnecting computers and magnetic tapes were method of transferring imaging information out of radiological scanners. Most radiological manufacturers are integrating Ethernet into their newer-generation scanners. *Fiber-distributed data interface* (FDDI) is an outgrowth of the refinement and improvement in fiber optic technology and is just beginning to be adopted on some computer networks. FDDI is many times faster than Ethernet.

Compact disk, read only memory (CD-ROM) was just beginning to appear in 1987. Today, entire encyclopedias are available on CD-ROM and many computer vendors are beginning to distribute their system software on CD-ROM. Write-once, ready many (WORM) and read-write *optical technology* are available today at a reasonable cost. Optical disks are appearing on most, if not all, new-generation radiological scanners as the archiving media.

Visualization is the processing of gaining insights from modeling and manipulating large multidimensional data sets. While a late 1980s buzzword, the process just describes what our group at Mayo Clinic has been doing in volumetric stereotaxis for years.

Virtual reality (VR) is a term that has gained much press recently. VR is computer-based simulator that currently utilizes gloves laced with sensors, stereo goggles, earphones or multidirectional sound and other props allowing one to simulate an imaginery virtual environment. Sensors track human motions and the virtual world is supposed to respond to them. Unfortunately, computing power and rendering software are not yet up to this challenge. Even with cartoon-like worlds, current VR systems often result in jerky movement of objects and delays in updating the virtual representation of the user's actions. Nevertheless, much of the development in VR may have impact on stereotactic neurosurgery in the future. For example, while one can today simulate a surgical procedure using a stereotactic treatment-planning system, one may be able to perform the simulated procedure on a computer-rendered and simulated virtual patient in the not too distant future.

Personal computing operating systems are just beginning to perform multitasking, whereby several programs or program steps seem to operate in unison even though only one is really running on the computer at one time. Today *distributed processing* relocates (distributes) computations at other computers over a network. The *X Windowing System* is perhaps one of the more exciting developments that may have impact on stereotactic neurosurgery. Developed at the Massachusetts Institute of Technology, X is being adopted as a standard network-based windowing system whereby an algorithm may run on a network of perhaps different vendor machines or be run on one machine and displayed on another somewhere on the network.

Future Trends

Many exciting new computing and imaging developments are on the horizon. Computers will continue to become faster and more capacious, but also will continue to integrate more information digitally (audio, video, film etc.). Some of the other new technologies that will become more mainstream in computing are *parallel processing* whereby hundreds, if not thousands, of processors will combine to perform calculations simultaneously. One hundred or more tiny lasers are being combined in what are currently known as Sarnoff chips, which are functional *optoelectric integrated circuits.* Furthermore, *quantum transistors* promise to be 100 times smaller and possible 1,000 times faster than today's transistors. *Superconductors* carrying electrical signals without loss of energy may prove useful in producing not only faster computing circuits but also more advanced radiological scanners.

Radiological manufacturers will continue to produce scanners with shorter scanning times, thinner slices and smaller pixel sizes. Furthermore, new-generation scanners will support true networking (rather than as an add-on) and multimodality imaging stations to view and quantitatively manipulate multiple images from multiple modalities at one location.

Networking technology will continue to improve providing faster networks not only on optical fiber, but also on wireless networks. Apple Computer has already petitioned the Federal Communications Commissions for a portion of the radio spectrum to be used for digital computing networks. The imaging workstation in every doctor's office or home is not too far away.

The future is bright for stereotactic neurosurgery. If Horsley and Clarke could only see what the field they pioneered has grown into!

Bruce A. Kall, MS, Mayo Clinic, 200 First ST, SW, 5-222 STM,
Rochester, MN 55905 (USA)

Proceedings of the Meeting of the American Society for Stereotactic and Functional Neurosurgery, Pittsburgh, Pa., June 16–19, 1991
Stereotact Funct Neurosurg 1992;58:94–98

Stereotactic Localization and Guidance Using a Machine Vision Technique

M. Peter Heilbrun, Paul McDonald, Clay Wiker, Spencer Koehler, William Peters

Division of Neurological Surgery, University of Utah School of Medicine, Salt Lake City, Utah, USA

Key Words. Stereotactic localization · Machine vision · Digitized video

Abstract. Machine vision techniques (video cameras) can be used to determine the three-dimensional position of objects. This transformation can be accomplished with standard mathematical algorithms. Initial accuracy tests of stereotactic localization with video cameras were performed using a standard Brown-Roberts-Wells (BRW) phantom simulator coupled with the BRW angiographic localizer. Localization accuracy was within 1.5 mm. Potential applications of machine vision techniques include freehand stereotactic localization of the position and orientation of surgical instruments. With sufficient computer speed these techniques can be used for continuous monitoring of the position of instruments within the cranial vault.

In a series of experiments to evaluate the accuracy of stereotactic coordinate systems defined with three-dimensional digitizers such as sonic digitizers, articulated arms and opticoelectrical digitizers, we noted than a machine vision technique using two video cameras could be used to define a stereotactic coordinate system. Our initial machine vision technique utilized radiographic perspective transformation with angiographic localizers like the ones designed by Gybels-Suetens and Siddon [1–4]. Instead of radiographic images, we substituted digitized video images of the fiduciary marks of the angiographic localizer. Once the concept was confirmed with a standard Brown-Roberts-Wells (BRW) angiographic localizer mated to a BRW phantom, we designed a new video projection localizer which ensured that all fiduciary marks could be seen on a video image outside the contour of the head.

1011–6125/92/0584–0094 $ 2.75/0

Table 1. Test of video-localizer-defined target compared to actual target and BRW-localizer-defined target

	Stereotactic coordinate		
	actual	BRW localizer	video localizer
Target test 1			
Anteroposterior	92.6	91.3	92.0
Lateral	–6.8	–6.5	–5.8
Vertical	14.0	14.9	13.2
Target test 2			
Anteroposterior	–16.0	–15.7	–17.8
Lateral	25.0	24.2	26.1
Vertical	48.4	48.1	48.4

Methods and Results

We have demonstrated the relative accuracy of the new video localizer using both a standard black-and-white video camera and a SuperVHS camcorder combined with high-resolution lens. By digitizing the images of the video localizer as they are captured by the two cameras placed from 40 to 60° apart, we attained accurate stereotactic coordinates within 2 mm of an actual stereotactic target (table 1). In addition, the cameras' zoom function enabled us to view the video localizer predominantly through the central portion of the lens, thereby avoiding pin cushion distortion of the image. We found that this localization technique could be accurate to 1.5 mm throughout a sphere of 40 cm which would encompass the head. We also demonstrated that, if the head and the two cameras remain in a fixed position throughout the procedure, the video localizer could be removed, and fiduciary marks attached to surgical instruments could be localized with the same cameras.

This machine vision technique coupled to our standard stereotactic computer system [5–7] makes possible freehand monitoring of the position of surgical instruments within a stereotactic coordinate system without requiring a specialized stereotactic guidance arc. Using standard geometric functions, we have also demonstrated that the tip of a surgical instrument within the cranium can be localized as long as the two fiduciary markers attached to the instrument can be seen simultaneously by the two video cameras.

Discussion

There are several advantages to a machine vision technique which defines a stereotactic coordinate system by video images of a projection type localizer instead of X-ray beams. Once the head (or other part of the body) is fixed in a standard operating room holding device (such as a Mayfield head pin or a stereotactic head ring), relatively inexpensive video cameras separated by a number of different angles and placed in many different positions define a stereotactic coordinate system. This machine vision stereotactic coordinate system can be mated with any accurately defined image coordinate system. Such a system can eliminate the burden of attaching a stereotactic arc or an articulated arm to a special head frame, or the necessary calibration to use a sonic digitizer. With low-cost PC-type computer systems equipped with dual frame grabbers, static localization of intracranial structures is easily accomplished. Using faster computers, real-time tracking of the position and orientation of instruments within the brain can be easily accomplished. In addition, combining machine vision techniques with ultrasound probes could accomplish relatively inexpensive real-time monitoring of intracranial structures within the same stereotactic coordinate system. Other machine vision techniques that use linear charged coupled devices (CCDs) to track both LEDs and reflected laser beams and grids in three dimensions are presently available commercially. We believe our system can be developed as a relatively simple system using off the shelf commodity components mated with presently available operating room head holders.

Disadvantages of the system are potential measurement inaccuracies from the video system including lens parallax, video pixel size and translation of the analog video signal to the a digital image. Such measurement problems are becoming less critical as the cost of linear CCDs decreases. These potential inaccuracies are presently being evaluated to determine the cost of a system with greater than 1 mm accuracy. Another disadvantage is the need to redefine the stereotactic coordinate system if the head fixation platform or the video cameras move.

Before the CT era, stereotactic localization was accomplished using fixed radiographic machines in the operating room. Direct visualization of intracranial and intraparenchymal structures became possible with the invention of CT scans. New stereotactic localization concepts were developed based on prospective imaging with a stereotactic reference platform fixed to the skull.

With the evolution of multiple image sets including CT, MRI and angiography for stereotactic localization, computer programs have been developed to cross-register these data sets by treating the image data sets as volume arrays. Analyzing these image data sets with advanced computer graphic techniques such as surface and volume rendering permits the correlation of external head and face landmarks to intracranial structures. This latter computer technique allows stereotactic localization of intracranial structures without fixation of a stereotactic reference frame preceding the surgical procedure, a method termed 'frameless stereotaxy' [8, 9]. In addition, we have developed computer programs to mate generically any image coordinate systems defined with cartesian coordinates to any stereotactic systems.

In conclusion, we have demonstrated the relative accuracy of using machine vision algorithms that are routinely used in the industrial work place to define a stereotactic coordinate system in the operating room. Combining this technology with computer systems that can mate cartesian image coordinate systems with stereotactic coordinate systems will allow neurosurgeons to make a transition from frame-based to frameless stereotactic techniques.

References

1 Siddon R, Barth N: Stereotaxic localization of intracranial targets. Int J Radiat Oncol Biol Phys 1987;13:1241–1246.

2 Suetens P, Gybels J, Jansen P, Oosterlinck A: A global 3-D image of the blood vessels, tumor, and simulated electrode. Acta Neurochir 1984;33:225–232.

3 Vandermeulen D, Suetens P, Gybels J: Angiographic localizer ring for the BRW stereotactic system. Acta Neurochir Suppl 1987;39:15–17.

4 Vandermeulen D, Suetens P, Gybels J, Oosterlinck A: A new software package for the microcomputer based BRW stereotactic system: Integrated stereoscopic views of CT data and angiograms. SPIE Med Image Processing 1985;593:103–104.

5 Bopp J, Krauss H: An orientation and calibration method for nontopographic applications. Photogrammetric Eng 1978;44:1191–1196.
6 Heilbrun M, Brown R, McDonald P: Real time three-dimensional graphic reconstructions using Brown-Roberts-Wells frame coordinates in a microcomputer environment. Appl Neurophysiol 1985;48:7–10.
7 Johnson H: The mechanical; engineer and the transition to image analysis. Adv Imaging 1990;5:52–56.
8 Freits E, Strobehn J, Hatch J, Roberts D: A frameless stereotactic operating microscope for neurosurgery. IEEE Trans Biomed Eng 1989;36:608–617.
9 Roberts D, Strohbehn J, Hatch J, Murray W, Kettenberger H: A frameless stereotaxic integration of computerized tomographic imaging and the operating microscope. J Neurosurg 1986;65:545–549.

M. Peter Heilbrun, MD, Division of Neurological Surgery,
University of Utah School of Medicine, 50 North Medical Dr. No. 3B406,
Salt Lake City, UT 84132 (USA)

Proceedings of the Meeting of the American Society for Stereotactic and Functional Neurosurgery, Pittsburgh, Pa., June 16–19, 1991
Stereotact Funct Neurosurg 1992;58:99–102

Utilization of Image-Derived Computer-Assisted Stereotaxis in a Community-Based Practice Setting

Chad D. Abernathey, Merilee Ramsey, Kathy Knight

Iowa Medical Clinic/Mercy Medical Center, Division of Neurosurgery, Cedar Rapids, Iowa, USA

Key Words. Stereotaxis · Stereotactic surgery · Computer · Stereotactic craniotomy

Abstract. The success of a community-based stereotactic program is dependent upon community commitment, technological capability, referral base, patient/family support and, most importantly, proper patient selection. To develop a program of superior quality requires not only a substantial financial commitment, but also a basic philosophical approach which fully supports acquisition and education of support staff, physical plant renovation and an establishment of an expanding referral base. This report details the development of a highly sophisticated stereotactic program in Cedar Rapids, Iowa, a semirural community with a base referral population of approximately 300,000.

Stereotactic computer-assisted laser microsurgery is well recognized among specialists in the field as a precise and accurate method of brain tumor localization and treatment. Having survived periods of varied popularity, stereotaxis has flourished in the past 10 years from its use in straightforward biopsy procedures to complete laser resection under computerized guidance and three-dimensional control [1–6]. Highly sophisticated technology of this nature, however, is generally situated within large university complexes or tertiary care centers. The program described herein was developed in a community-based clinical practice setting and has demonstrated remarkable success in regard to utilization and clinical results.

The success of a community-based stereotactic program is dependent upon several integrated factors. These include community com-

1011–6125/92/0584–0099 $ 2.75/0

Table 1. Stereotactic procedures performed from November 1989 to May 1991 in a community-based practice setting

Operative procedure	n
Craniotomy for tumor	24
Biopsy	10
Abscess drainage	1
Cyst drainage/Ommaya reservoir placement for P32 installation	1
Colloid cyst excision	1
Ventriculoscopic fenestration of cavum septum pellucidum cyst with wick placement	1
Excision radiation necrosis	1
Resection of cavernous angioma	1

mitment related to financial support for equipment acquisition and physical plant renovation of the designated site. It also demands recruitment of medical staff and ongoing education of essential support staff. Finally, it is essential to develop a referral base that is large enough to maintain the economic viability of the program. Creating an awareness of services among the medical as well as lay community via a discrete but effective marketing plan is key in the development of such a referral base.

Materials and Methods

Mercy Medical Center (MMC) is a 350-bed private, not-for-profit acute care hospital in Cedar Rapids, Iowa, a city with a population of approximately 110,000. In the spring of 1989, MMC made a commitment to create a stereotactic program in consultation and cooperation with a private neurosurgical practice. The project was funded with MMC endowment funds and is a key component of the center's expanding neuroscience services.

Results

Our experience to date in Cedar Rapids, Iowa (November 1989–May 1991), has included 38 patients undergoing 40 volumetric computer-assisted stereotactic procedures in a community-based clinical prac-

Table 2. Pathologic findings for 40 consecutive stereotactic procedures in a community-based practice setting

Lesion pathology	n
High-grade astrocytoma (III–IV)	12
Metastatic	9
Recurrent astrocytoma	4
Meningioma	2
Demyelinating plaque	2
Radiation necrosis	2
Low-grade astrocytoma (I–II)	2
Abscess	1
Colloid cyst	1
Cavum septum pellucidum cyst	1
Infarct	1
Osteoma	1
Cavernous angioma	1

tice setting. Patient age has ranged from 28 to 78 years, including 24 males and 14 females. Most cases presented with sensorimotor deficits of seizures. Two were incidental findings on imaging studies after trauma.

38 procedures were performed for supratentorial pathology. Two posterior fossa procedures utilized a unique software program requiring inversion of the head frame. Table 1 displays the data for operative techniques employed. Table 2 demonstrates the lesion pathology encountered (note: 2 cases included recurrence of original diagnosis). No operative complications were identified, as all patients tolerated the procedures well. Notably, no new deficits or significant hemorrhages occurred. All patients improved neurologically or had normal examinations following the craniotomy procedures. Biopsy patients were essentially unchanged from their preoperative status. Proper localization of the surgical site was confirmed and resection margins assessed with postoperative imaging in all cases. Average perioperative hospitalization was 2 days for non-craniotomy procedures and 4.5 days for craniotomy cases.

Conclusion

Sophisticated 'high-tech' equipment, regardless of the practice setting, does not stand alone. A dedicated and motivated medical staff in conjunction with a well-coordinated team of surgical, radiological and nursing personnel ensures a facile orchestration of each individualized stereotactic procedure. Practice sessions with the designated OR team allow for hands-on equipment assembly and room preparation. Structured lectures including a review of pertinent anatomy, specific procedural details, and pre-, intra- and postoperative protocols were developed to ensure a thorough knowledge of the procedure and to provide consistency in care. Our experience demonstrates that sophisticated volumetric computer-assisted image-guided stereotactic systems can be applied to a community-based clinical practice setting to enhance the scope of services, as well as provide for safe and reliable, diagnostic and therapeutic intracranial techniques.

References

1 Abernathey CD, Camacho A, Kelly PJ: Stereotaxic suboccipital transcerebellar biopsy of pontine mass lesions. J Neurosurg 1989;70:195–200.
2 Abernathey CD, Davis DH, Kelly PJ: Management of colloid cysts by stereotactic microsurgical craniotomy. J Neurosurg 1989;70:525–529.
3 Abernathey CD, Kelly PJ: Computer assisted stereotactic laser microsurgery. Lasers Med Sci 1988;3:365.
4 Kelly PJ: Computerized guidance for stereotactic treatment of brain tumors. Neurosurgery 1987;2:165–191.
5 Kelly PJ, Kall BA, Goerss SJ, et al: Results of computer assisted stereotactic laser resection of deep-seated intracranial lesions. Mayo Clin Proc 1986;61:20–27.
6 Kelly PJ, et al.: Imaging based stereotactic serial biopsies in untreated intracranial glial neoplasms. J Neurosurg 1987;66:865–874.

Chad D. Abernathey, MD, 1519 Center Point Rd., NE, Cedar Rapids, IA 52402 (USA)

Proceedings of the Meeting of the American Society for Stereotactic and Functional Neurosurgery, Pittsburgh, Pa., June 16–19, 1991
Stereotact Funct Neurosurg 1992;58:103–107

An Independent Application Accuracy Evaluation of Stereotactic Frame Systems

Robert J. Maciunas, Robert L. Galloway, Jr., Jim Latimer, Charles Cobb, Eric Zaccharias, Andrew Moore, Venkat R. Mandava

Departments of Neurological Surgery and Biomedical Engineering, Vanderbilt University Medical Center, Nashville, Tenn., USA

Key Words. Stereotactic · Accuracy · Precision · Stereotactic frame · Imaging · CT

Abstract. The purpose of incorporating stereotactic methodology into neurosurgical procedures is to consistently achieve a high degree of accuracy and precision in localizing intracranial targets. Therefore, the limits of resolution for the therapeutic intervention itself are a function of the accuracy and precision inherent to the particular stereotactic frame system itself. The total clinically relevant error (application accuracy) comprises errors associated with each procedural step, including imaging, target selection, vector calculation and the mechanical errors of stereotactic frames. To evaluate these parameters, a systematic error analysis was carried out in the 4 most commonly used CT-compatible stereotactic devices: the Brown-Roberts-Wells, Cosman-Roberts-Wells, Kelly-Goerss Compass (modified Todd-Wells) and Leksell frames. Over 7,681 independent test measurements were made. The results suggest a potentially significant degree of error in application accuracy of all stereotactic instrumentation which is accentuated by imaging-associated error. These individual error values must be considered with every clinical use of stereotactic frames.

Stereotactic instrumentation and methodology were described in 1908 by Horsley and Clarke [1]. Subsequently, numerous technical advances brought about by many investigators have resulted in a clinically significant addition to the neurosurgical armamentarium for procedures requiring accurate and precise intraoperative localization. Stereotactic methodology has been applied successfully to the direction of electrode implantation, radioisotope implantation, radiosurgery, biopsy, resection and ablation, among many other procedures.

The rationale for applying stereotactic methodology to neurosurgical procedures is to access targets with a minimum of spatial error (i.e.,

1011–6125/92/0584–0103 $ 2.75/0

high *accuracy*) and a high degree of reproducibility (i.e., high *precision*). The clinical reliance upon stereotactic instrumentation to provide accurate target localization requires that a quantitative basis exist for this degree of trust. Previously published evaluations of stereotactic instruments, however, have not conclusively dealt with this issue. Limitations of previous literature include inadequate sample size for statistical analysis, failure to control for variables introduced by imaging techniques, artificially constrained testing conditions such as target points located only at the center of the imaging field or the use of approach trajectories that minimize machining errors of the instruments, and reliance upon purely clinical criteria for success of localization [2].

In addition to the mechanical limitations of the stereotactic frames, the error associated with the many steps of stereotaxy (including imaging techniques, point selection and vector calculation) all contribute to the final clinically relevant error. The purpose of this study is to go beyond assessment of the *mechanical accuracy* of various stereotactic frames to assess what has been called the *application accuracy* [2] or accuracy of the devices as used in a real-world setting. This is separate and distinct from any measure of *precision* associated with the machinery of the stereotactic frame construction itself.

Methods

Application accuracy was assessed in the 4 most commonly used stereotactic frames, using methods similar to those used for stereotactic neurosurgery. The frame systems tested were the *Brown-Roberts-Wells* (BRW) and *Cosman-Roberts-Wells* (CRW; Radionics, Burlington, Mass., USA), the *Kelly-Goerss (modified Todd-Wells)* (Stereotactic Medical Systems, New Hartford, N.Y., USA) and the *Leksell* (Elekta Instruments, Tucker, Ga., USA).

Test phantoms were developed which consisted of radiodense carbon fiber targets fixed to one end of rigid acrylic plastic rods of different heights; the non-target ends of the rods were embedded orthogonally in a random pattern in a base of acrylic plastic.

The stereotactic frame was affixed to the phantom base, and the apparatus was imaged via a Siemens Somatom DR-H-type CT scanner. For each apparatus, multiple imaging runs were made with different slice thicknesses and slice planes. For each run, the apparatus was scanned successively from the base to the most distal target. Runs with slices of 1, 4 and 8 mm were made in the plane perpendicular to the rods. One-millimeter slices in a plane at a canted angle to the N bars were also taken to assess the robustness of the localization algorithm with regard to frame orientation. The CT slices were carefully selected to cut precisely through the tips of the targets in the 1-mm straight and canted CT views, to provide an optimized situation of ideal localization.

Table 1. Results of application accuracy evaluation of 4 representative stereotactic frame systems (7,681 total independent accuracy measurements)

CT slice thickness	Measurement, mm			
	BRW	CRW	Kelly-Goerss	Leksell
Phantom base (mechanical accuracy)				
Mean	0.6	0.7	NA	NA
SD	0.4	0.4		
Max. value	3.1	5.0		
99% CL	1.8	2.0		
1 mm				
Mean	1.9	1.8	1.0	1.7
SD	1.0	1.1	0.6	1.0
Max. value	5.0	4.9	3.1	4.5
99% CL	4.8	5.1	2.7	4.6
1 mm canted (angulation effect)				
Mean	2.5	2.2	1.5	NA
SD	1.1	1.1	1.0	
Max. value	6.9	6.1	5.0	
99% CL	5.9	5.7	4.3	
4 mm				
Mean	2.7	2.6	2.5	3.2
SD	1.3	1.5	1.4	1.3
Max. value	7.0	7.1	6.2	5.2
99% CL	6.6	7.1	6.8	7.2
8 mm				
Mean	6.6	6.6	5.1	5.3
SD	3.1	3.0	2.9	2.4
Max. value	11.2	12.0	10.9	10.2
99% CL	15.8	15.7	13.8	12.6

SD = Standard deviation; Max. = maximal value; CL = confidence level; NA = not assessed.

The 4- and 8-mm slices were obtained in standard clinical imaging protocol technique, without a priori centering upon the target tips, so as to more realistically reproduce clinically relevant localization protocols. The spatial locations of the fiducial marks and target points were extracted from the CT images using standard protocols for each frame system.

For each target point, frame settings for 3 approach trajectories were calculated using the localization algorithm supplied by the frame manufacturer. The stereotactic localization arc was then attached to the frame, and a measuring probe was introduced to the appropriate depth. The distance from the tip of the probe to the tip of the target was measured as the application error. This testing was carried out for *multiple* frames of *each type* of stereotactic instrument, with no less than *five* independent trials at each point, with *multiple* trajectories, with *multiple* CT scans. The mechanical error of *multiple* BRW/CRW stereotactic phantom bases was independently tested in a similar fashion.

Results and Conclusions

Table 1 details the results of over 7,681 independent trials for assessment of application accuracy of the 4 representative stereotactic frame systems.

The application accuracy of the 4 most commonly used stereotactic frame systems is less than the mechanical accuracy and precision described for these systems. Any differences in application accuracy between the 4 stereotactic frame systems tested are less significant than the differences in application accuracy between individual target localizations using CT scans of differing slice thicknesses.

The level of localization error noted in trials using CT scan slice thicknesses of 8 mm suggests that satisfactory stereotactic localization of smaller intracranial targets requires thinner CT scan slices. Localization of a CT-defined target using orthogonally oriented 1-mm-thick scan slices centered upon that target represents an optimized situation. Using currently available stereotactic instrumentation, the 99% confidence levels for accuracy of target localization in this ideal case are in the range of 3.0–5.1 mm. This error is greater than that attributable to imaging error, being larger than the dimensions of a voxel.

These results must be kept in mind by the clinician in planning each surgery employing stereotactic instrumentation and methodology, so as to tailor an optimal image acquisition protocol for an appropriate confidence level in target localization during that individual therapeutic intervention.

References

1 Horsley V, Clarke RH: The structure and functions of the cerebellum examined by a new method. Brain 1908;31:45.
2 Galloway RL, Maciunas RJ: Stereotactic neurosurgery. CRC Crit Rev Biomed Eng 1990;18:181–205.

Robert J. Maciunas, MD, Department of Neurological Surgery, T 4224 MCN, Vanderbilt University Medical Center, Nashville, TN 37232 (USA)

Proceedings of the Meeting of the American Society for Stereotactic and Functional Neurosurgery, Pittsburgh, Pa., June 16–19, 1991
Stereotact Funct Neurosurg 1992;58:108–113

A Universal System for Interactive Image-Directed Neurosurgery

Robert J. Maciunas, Robert L. Galloway, Jr., J. Michael Fitzpatrick, Venkat R. Mandava, Charles A. Edwards, George S. Allen

Departments of Neurological Surgery, Biomedical Engineering and Computer Science, Vanderbilt University Medical Center, Nashville, Tenn., USA

Key Words. Stereotactic · Computer · Localizing arm · Neurosurgery, image-directed

Abstract. Stereotactic methods confer great accuracy to intracranial target localization, but require strict adherence to a complex program of mechanical and computational maneuvers. A computerized, articulated, localizing 'arm' has been developed that frees the neurosurgeon of these constraints and provides a completely intuitive, 'user-friendly' interface. This universal system is independent of whatever localizing fiducial system is selected. The arm may be sterilized for intracranial use. A variety of intraoperative end effectors may be selected. The patient's CT/MR/PET scans are loaded into computer memory and a three-dimensional shaded surface wireframe diagram of the patient's head is displayed simultaneously with up to 3 independent sets of cross-referenced CT/MR/PET scan images on the intraoperative video screen. The arm's endpoint location and the directional vector are shown as cursors on the relevant scan slices, and change continuously as the surgeon moves the arm. Because the information is continuously updated, an unlimited number of targets and trajectories may be displayed throughout the operation. The arm has an ultimate design accuracy for endpoint localization to within 0.1 mm throughout a target volume of 40 × 40 × 40 cm. The tested application accuracy of the first prototype model is 0.31 mm. In clinical use during 30 surgeries, its real-world application accuracy is 0.9 mm. This system provides stereotactic accuracy and universally compatible, intuitive, interactive operation.

Introduction

Interactive image-directed (IID) surgery is a derivative of stereotactic surgery. The term stereotactic arises from stereo, for three-dimensional, and tactus, to touch, and thus would apply to IID surgery as well. In medical practice, however, stereotactic surgery has come to mean the use of an external framework and a rigid vernier-based guid-

1011–6125/92/0584–0108 $ 2.75/0

ance arc assembly attached to the patient to allow geometrically determined vectors to internal surgical points of interest. These vectors are determined by making measurements from the images, performing calculations based on those measurements and positioning the arc assembly verniers so that it may direct a probe or retractor system along the desired trajectory. We distinguish IID surgery from traditional arc-directed stereotactic surgery in that IID surgery allows interactive and intuitive freedom of choice for both targets and trajectories throughout surgery.

IID surgery is the next step for utilization of concepts developed in stereotactic surgery devices. Technological advances over the past 4 years in angular sensing, desktop computer speeds and high-speed raster displays have made IID a real possibility. Initial design work, prototype construction and computer simulations show that an IID system is feasible with present technology and for a reasonable cost.

Articulated Localizing Arm

The arm is a 3-link, 3-joint, 6-degree-of-freedom articulated stainless-steel arm. Each joint consists of two rotational angles, mounted in a gimbal structure. This configuration leads to 330° of free motion in each joint.

The angular sensors are incremental 16-bit optical encoders that interpolate 72,000 pulses per rotation. Optical encoders give improved linearity, better resolution and reduced sensitivity to environmental factors, such as temperature.

The angular position is transmitted to the angular sensors via spur gears, which are oriented to minimize backlash. The joint bearings are preloaded, minimizing unmeasured lateral motion in each joint. The arm construction permits gas sterilization of the entire arm assembly. The end effector is replaceable in order to hold other medical devices such as dissectors, suckers, shunt tubes, lasers, ultrasound transducers or electrodes.

Intraoperative Scan Image Video Display

Our display technique uses numerical data from the scanner's tapes, not film-and-video capture. Four fully 512 × 512 pixel image win-

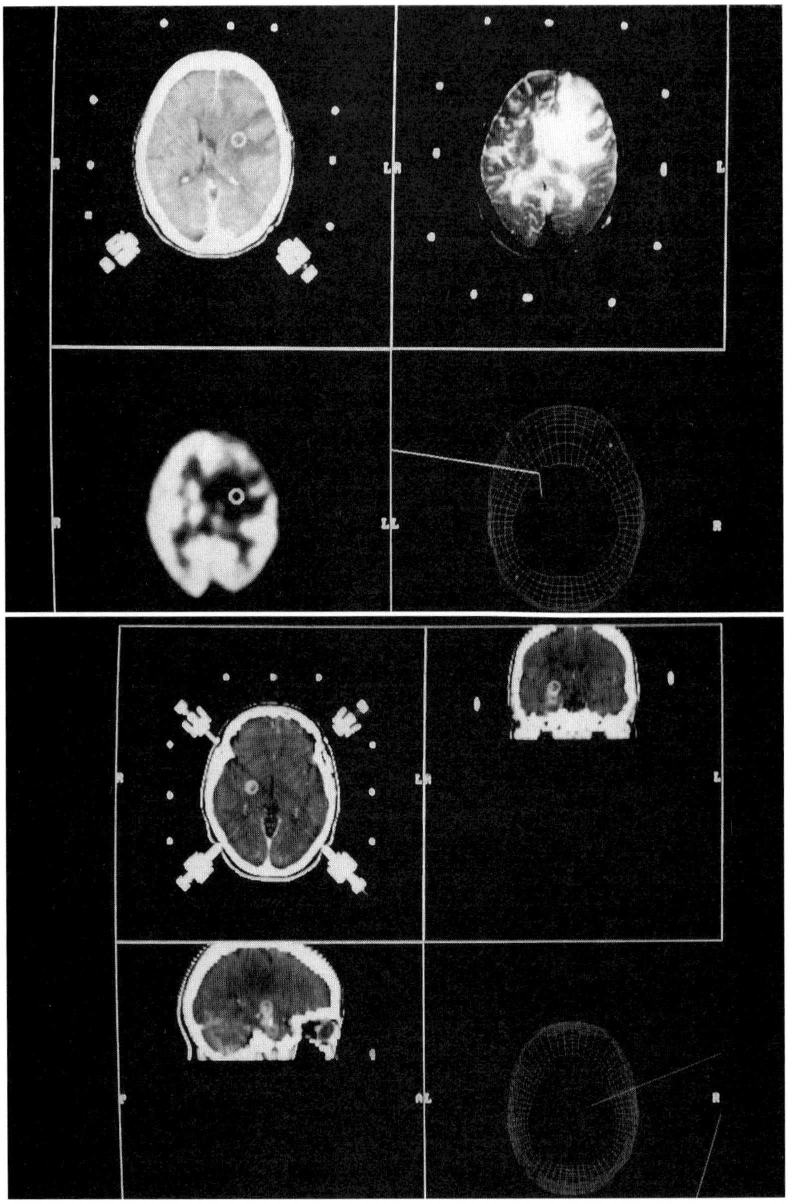

a

b

Fig. 1. Computer video displays of intraoperative arm position relative to correlated CT, MR and PET scans (**a**) during biopsy and (**b**) relative to axial, coronal and sagittal reformated CT images during craniotomy.

dows prevent degradation of image resolution. When motion occurs out of the present slice, the new slice is displayed where the old one was. This means, for example, that pure motion in the z direction is shown as a stationary x-y cursor position with a new displayed image. Thus, there is no searching for cursor location. Finally, we provide a patient-specific, perspective, graphic display to help with orientation and visualization. The raster images are used for targeting, and the graphics images are used for three-dimensional orientation and trajectory information.

Display of three-dimensional information can take several forms: (1) display of the closest slice as determined by the endpoint position; (2) 'reslicing' of the imaging volume to display a new slice perpendicular to the arm position vector, or (3) pseudo-three-dimensional displays, using ray projection and variable opacity techniques or wireframe projections. In this prototype, we have opted for the simplest raster display, which is the x and y position display on the closest z slice, and have coupled this image registration with the simplest graphic display, a wireframe.

Computational Hardware Configuration

An 80386-based computer system is presently being used as the computational platform for this initial system. With the inclusion of a math co-processor, the computer has a rating of approximately 0.5 MFlop. The images are stored in the computer on a 383M hard disk (CDC Wren 5) and can be read from the disk and displayed in less than a third of a second. This assures real-time video display rates.

A Matrox PG-1281 color display adaptor handles the image display. With a BITBLT rate of 100 million bits/second (12.5 million 8 bit pixels), it can place a new 512 × 512 image on the screen every 21 ms.

Our display technique uses numerical data from the scanner's tapes, not film-and-video capture. A 9-in tape drive is currently configured to allow direct scanner-to-surgical planning/intraoperative system transfer of image data and header file information. Three fully 512 × 512 pixel image windows prevent degradation of image resolution.

The display is composed of three 512 × 512 gray-scale windows displaying images from modalities such as CT/MR/PET and one 512 × 512 graphics window presently showing a patient-specific wireframe model

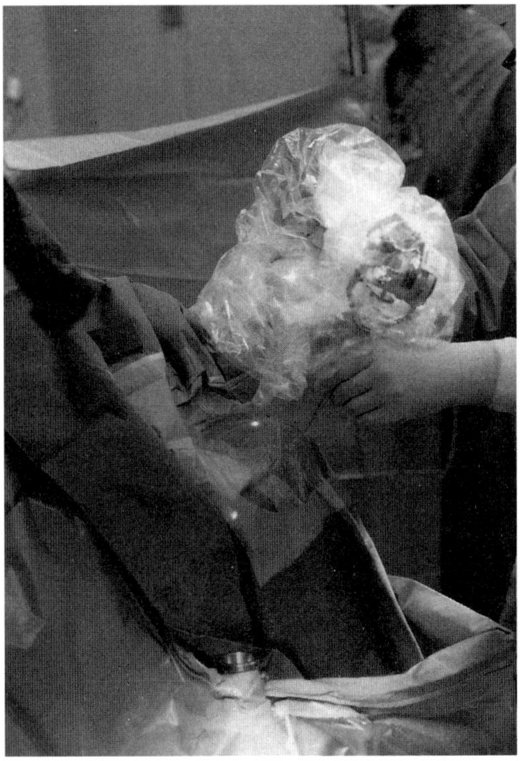

Fig. 2. Intraoperative localizing arm.

(fig. 1). The display was initially accomplished by compressing the raster image (CT, MRI, PET) to 240 gray levels and using the remaining 16 colors for the graphics display. A new display device now allows true 12-bit display (CT, MRI, PET standard) with 4 bits of overlay for graphic models.

Testing of Articulated Arm

Precision Testing

The arm precision was tested by picking an arbitrary point within the volume the arm can reach. The point was located by touching the arm to the point and then brought back to the point in an arbitrary, but different path. The standard deviation of the distance measurements was 0.27 mm.

Accuracy Testing

In order to make appropriate accuracy measurements, the three-dimensional relationships of the structures within a phantom were measured using electronic calipers. Points within the phantom were measured with the arm and compared to the caliper measurements. The arm was able to locate a point to a mean error of 0.31 mm.

Clinical Trials

This system has been used for intraoperative localization during 30 cases to date: 20 craniotomies and 10 biopsies (fig. 2). The IID system has consistently been within 1 pixel of the localization by traditional frame and arc stereotactic systems.

The real-world application accuracy of localization for this system during surgery has proven to be less than 0.9 mm.

References

1 Galloway RL, Maciunas RJ: Stereotactic neurosurgery. CRC Crit Rev Biomed Eng 1990;18:181–205.

2 Balogh AE, Springfield J, Maciunas RJ, Galloway RL: Simulation and error analysis for a stereotactic pointing system. Proc Annu Int Conf IEEE Eng Med Biol Soc, Nov 1989, vol 11, p 925.

3 Galloway RL, Edwards CA, Haden GL, Maciunas RJ: Creation of a wire-frame model for three-dimensional registration of raster image regions of interest. Proc SPIE, Medical Imaging IV. Newport Beach, Feb 1990, vol 1232, p 371.

4 Galloway RL, Edwards C, Haden GL, Maciunas RJ: A three-dimensional locator for stereotactic neurosurgery. Proc Annu Int Conf IEEE Eng Med Biol Soc, Nov 1989, vol 11, p 1935.

Robert J. Maciunas, MD, Department of Neurological Surgery, T 4224 MCN, Vanderbilt University Medical Center, Nashville, TN 37232 (USA)

Proceedings of the Meeting of the American Society for Stereotactic and Functional Neurosurgery, Pittsburgh, Pa., June 16–19, 1991
Stereotact Funct Neurosurg 1992;58:114–117

Further Development and Clinical Application of the Stereotactic Operating Microscope[1]

David W. Roberts, Taku Nakajima, Brian Brodwater, John Pavlidis, Eric Friets, Erin Fagan, Alex Hartov, John Strohbehn

Section of Neurosurgery, Dartmouth Medical School, and Thayer School of Engineering, Dartmouth College, Hanover, N.H., USA

Key Words. Stereotactic surgery · Frameless stereotaxy · Extracranial stereotaxy · Operating microscope

Abstract. Implementation of a Vicom-VME image processing workstation for the frameless stereotactic operating microscope system has allowed an improved interpolation algorithm for more accurate reconstruction of three-dimensional data, the integration graphically of multimodality imaging information, an additional stereotactic graphics display outside of the microscope optics and optional three-dimensional displays through communication with a Convex mini-supercomputer. A precision-milled coupling for reproducible attachment of the spark gap bracket to the microscope has eliminated the need for that transformation calculation during each case. Clinical utility has been greatest in providing navigational guidance to small subcortical or deep lesions and in defining the extent of preoperatively planned resection of larger, infiltrating tumors. Mean accuracy in the past 17 cases has been 3.5–6.5 mm. The frameless methodology has also enabled extracranial stereotactic surgical procedures in 7 patients.

The concept of a computer-based stereotactic operating microscope system, by which CT and MRI data can be spatially registered with the operative field via the optics of a freely movable microscope, has been previously demonstrated in a working prototype [1–4]. Progress in the further development of this system is reviewed in terms of computer hardware, software capability, digitizer and registration refinement, and clinical utilization.

[1] Supported in part by DHHS/NIH grant GM37308.

1011–6125/92/0584–0114 $ 2.75/0

Table 1. Intracranial stereotactic operating microscope cases (January 1990–June 1991)

Patient No.	Pathology	Handheld check, mm	Focal point check, mm		
			total	depth	inplane
1	meningioma	7.17			
2	metastasis	0.78			
3	glioma	5.59			
4	glioma	3.78			
5	glioma	3.40			
6	metastasis	7.07			
7	meningioma	1.51	7.00	4.50	5.40
8	meningioma	4.09	12.55	6.95	10.01
9	glioma	2.34	8.09	2.18	7.68
10	metastasis	3.74	10.65	8.45	6.28
11	metastasis	2.69	3.31	2.66	1.81
12	meningioma	2.87	3.04	2.16	2.14
13	meningioma	4.42	7.30	1.28	6.97
14	metastasis	2.04	8.62	3.20	7.87
15	glioma	2.86	3.24	0.71	3.16
16	cavernous angioma	1.96	1.29	1.04	0.76
17	choroid plexus cyst	1.15	4.60	3.00	3.49
Mean		3.38	6.33	3.28	5.05
SD		1.81	3.37	2.34	2.83

Materials and Methods

To enable further development, entirely rewritten system software has been implemented on a Vicom-VME image-processing workstation (consisting of a Sun 3/160 microcomputer with an enhanced backplane of image-processing hardware). Conversion from the IBM personal computer to the Vicom workstation has allowed an improved interpolation algorithm for more accurate reconstruction of three-dimensional data, the addition of angiographic information to the patient data base, integration graphically of multimodality imaging information and an additional stereotactic graphics display outside of the microscope optics. Display of three-dimensional contours, either as a stack of parallel outline images or as triangulated volumes, is possible through Ethernet communication with a Convex mini-supercomputer. A precision-milled coupling for reproducible attachment of the spark gap bracket to the microscope has eliminated the need for calculation of this transformation for each operative case, further facilitating and shortening the registration procedure.

Accuracy of the system during operative procedures has been evaluated using an additional fiducial point not used in the initial registration step. Image acquisition and

Table 2. Extracranial stereotactic operating microscope cases (January 1990–June 1991)

Patient No.	Pathology	Handheld check, mm	Inplane focal point check, mm	Disk space check, mm
1	HNP L3–4	3.10		26.23
2	HNP L5–S1	3.91		
3	HNP L4–5	3.44		23.65
4	HNP L5–S1	2.49	6.76	29.99
5	spondylolisthesis	3.98	11.47	22.92
6	HNP L5–S1	2.77	3.30	
7	HNP L5–S1		2.65	41.27
Mean		3.28	6.04	28.81
SD		0.55	3.50	5.96

HNP = Herniated nucleus pulposus.

processing, spatial registration in the operating room and preliminary performance of the digitizer are assessed by placement of a handheld spark gap at the independent fourth fiducial. Performance of the system in its entirety is assessed by positioning of the microscope focal point on that fiducial and measurement of the distance (expressed in terms of total distance, distance from the focal plane to the fiducial, and distance between the focal point and the fiducial's projection onto the focal plane) between the calculated position of the focal point and the known position of the fiducial. Evaluation of the system intraoperatively in terms of clinical utility, which is inherently more subjective, has been performed across a variety of tumor, vascular and other procedures. In addition, the system has been employed during surgical procedures involving the lumbosacral spine, using the same methodology of fiducial registration.

Results

Since implementation of the above system changes, the stereotactic operating microscope has been used in 17 intracranial cases (5 malignant glioma, 5 metastatic tumor, 5 meningioma, 1 cyst of the lateral ventricular choroid plexus and 1 cavernous angioma). Accuracy data for these cases is provided in table 1. Mean handheld check error was 3.38 mm (SD 1.81 mm), and mean focal point error was 6.33 mm (total), 3.28 mm (depth) and 5.05 mm (inplane).

Seven extracranial cases (6 lumbar herniated nucleus pulposus and 1 lumbar spondylolysis with spondylolisthesis) have been operated upon using the system, and accuracy data for these is shown in table 2. Mean handheld check for these was 3.28 mm (SD 0.55 mm); mean inplane system error was 6.04 mm.

Discussion

The system's greatest clinical utility has been in providing navigational assistance to small subcortical or deep lesions and in defining the extent of preoperatively planned resection of large infiltrative lesions. Frameless stereotactic methods enable potentially useful extracranial application, although tissue deformations render poorer accuracy at this time; more sophisticated correction algorithms or real-time imaging feedback may be beneficial in this regard. The system's currently less optimal attributes with respect to ease of use, speed and accuracy have been outweighed by the capabilities it provides and are all resolvable through the implementation of available technology.

References

1 Hatch JF, Roberts DW, Strohbehn JW: Reference-display system for the integration of CT scanning and the operating microscope; in Kulinski WS, Ohley WJ (eds): Proceedings of the 11th Annual Northeast Bioenginering Conference. New York, IEEE, 1985, pp 252–254.

2 Roberts DW, Strohbehn JW, Hatch JF, Murray W, Kettenberger H: A frameless stereotaxic integration of computerized tomographic imaging and the operating microscope. J Neurosurg 1986;65:545–549.

3 Friets EM, Strohbehn JW; Hatch JF, Roberts DW: A frameless stereotaxic operating microscope for neurosurgery. IEEE Trans Biomed Eng 1989;36:608–617.

4 Roberts DW, Strohbehn JW, Friets EM, Kettenberger J, Hartov A: The stereotactic operating microscope: Accuracy refinement and clinical experience. Acta Neurochir 1989(suppl 46):112–114.

D.W. Roberts, Section of Neurosurgery, Dartmouth-Hitchcock Medical Center, Hanover, NH 03756 (USA)

Proceedings of the Meeting of the American Society for Stereotactic and Functional Neurosurgery, Pittsburgh, Pa., June 16–19, 1991
Stereotact Funct Neurosurg 1992;58:118–120

Stereotactic Magnetic Resonance Angiography

Gene H. Barnett, Donald W. Kormos, Charles P. Steiner

Center for Computer Assisted Neurosurgery, Department of Neurosurgery, Cleveland Clinic Foundation, One Clinic Center, Cleveland, Ohio, USA

Key Words. Stereotactic techniques · Magnetic resonance angiography · Stereotactic biopsy · Depth electrodes

Abstract. Visualization of the surgical trajectory with respect to the cerebral vasculature may enhance the safety of some stereotactic neurosurgical procedures. Traditional stereotactic angiography is tedious and, being an invasive procedure, poses some risk to the patient. A technique of projecting a stereotactically defined surgical trajectory onto magnetic resonance angiograms is presented.

The development of computer image-guided stereotactic techniques has led to the widespread use of stereotactically guided biopsy and craniotomy. Although CT- and MRI-guided techniques enhance surgical planning, they provide little, if any, information on the cerebrovasculature along the surgical trajectory. Preoperative knowledge of the relationship of vessels, both arterial and venous, to the targest structure along the surgical trajectory, and on the cerebral surface (particularly for twist drill procedures), should reduce the risk of patient morbidity due to hemorrhage (fig. 1). Traditional stereotactic angiography is invasive, carries a small but appreciable risk of stroke, may require overnight hospitalization and can provide only limited viewing angles after data acquisition in a pseudo-three-dimensional fashion. Application of stereotactic techniques to magnetic resonance angiography (MRA) offers the potential advantages of being noninvasive, having no known risk, being an outpatient procedure, and allowing for true three-dimensional (3-D) visualization of the vascular tree and the surgical trajectory from any viewing angle after data acquisition. Our present approach to developing stereotactic MRA is presented.

1011–6125/92/0584–0118 $ 2.75/0

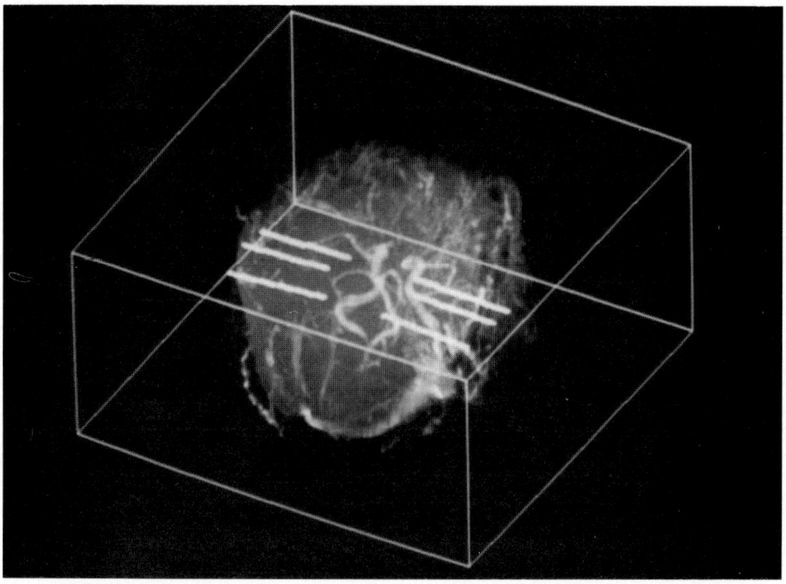

Fig. 1. Stereotactic MRA with projected trajectories of bilateral temporal lobe depth electrodes.

Methods

After conventional CT localization, a Compass™ (Stereotactic Medical Systems, Rochester, Minn., USA) MR localizer is applied to the patient's head in the usual fashion. A Siemens 1.5-tesla Magnetom SP is utilized for stereotactic MR localization. At the end of the MR study, a 3-D FISP time-of-flight, flow acquisition is performed, providing 64 (128) slices of MRA data in about 10 (20) min. The resulting flow-encoded images are transferred to a Sun Microsystems 4/370 workstation, the host computer for the Sun/Vicom Compass system, for preprocessing. Although images can be transferred on 0.5-in magnetic tape at a density of 1,600 bpi, typically, the images are transferred using an Ethernet channel implemented on a clinic-wide, local area network. Sun Microsystem' SunLink DNI software provides network connectivity between the Siemens host computer (Digital Equipment MicroVax) and the Sun 4/370 computer. Images are transferred at a rate of approximately 1 image per second. The Sun 4/370 is equipped with 32 megabytes of RAM and has 2.1 gigabytes of SCSI disk space. Preprocessing steps include stripping the images of header information, scaling and combination into a single 3-D MRA data file. Individual images are suitable for Compass stereotactic software. The 3-D data file is transferred over the network to a Stardent 3040 graphics supercomputer. Two-point trajectories are planned using the standard Compass software on the Sun workstation. The Compass target and entry points may then be automatically extracted from the surgical plan or manually entered into the Stardent for use with the 3-D data. The Stardent uses a modified maximum intensity pixel processing scheme to create the MRA projective images. Selected images (axial, coronal, sagittal, trajectory view) are ported back over the network to the Sun/Vicom hardware. Standard Compass software is then used to visualize the stereotactic MRA images along with the traditional CT and MR scans.

Discussion

Our present work demonstrates that stereotactic MRA is technically feasible, although issues of spatial fidelity remain. Unlike CT where spatial fidelity is dictated by the geometric configuration and mechanical alignment of its detectors, MRI and MRA presume linear field gradients throughout the imaged volume. Field inhomogeneities due either to aberrations of the imager itself, magnetic susceptibility effects or ferromagnetic effects from the patient and/or the localizer can produce appreciable local spatial distortions in the image. Approaches to rectify this problem include correlation with CT vasculature with appropriate re-registration of the MRA in stereotactic space.

Although the cost of the equipment used in this pilot project is considerable, the cost of equipment with comparable computational abilities is plummeting. It is conceivable that, within a few years, computers capable of such feats may cost no more than contemporary advanced personal computers.

Gene H. Barnett, MD, The Center for Computer Assisted Neurosurgery, Department of Neurosurgery, Cleveland Clinic Foundation, One Clinic Center, Cleveland, OH 44195 (USA)

Proceedings of the Meeting of the American Society for Stereotactic and Functional Neurosurgery, Pittsburgh, Pa., June 16–19, 1991
Stereotact Funct Neurosurg 1992;58:121–133

In vivo and in vitro Study of the Lesions Produced with a Computerized Radiofrequency System

F.C. Vinas[a], *L. Zamorano*[b], *M. Dujovny*[a], *J.Z. Zhao*[a], *D. Hodgkinson*[a], *K.L. Ho*[a], *J.I. Ausman*[a]

[a] Henry Ford Neurosurgical Institute Detroit, Mich.,
[b] Department of Neurosurgery, University Health Center, Wayne State University, Detroit, Mich., USA

Key Words. Stereotactic surgery · Radiofrequency · Functional neurosurgery · Lesion · Electrodes

Abstract. For many years, radiofrequency-generated lesions have been used for the treatment of pain and abnormal movements. However, the reliability of this method has been questioned because of the variation in the size of lesions produced by the electrode at different times and temperatures. A 500-kHz radiofrequency generator with different electrodes was used to determine the size of lesions, using different time and temperature exposures. A computerized feedback mechanism kept the tip temperature constant during the production of the lesion, regardless of varying tissue impedance. Eight electrodes of different size and tip characteristics were evaluated at different temperatures and time settings, both in vitro and in vivo. Graphic display of the curves in time were obtained at 65, 70, 75, 80, 85 and 90 °C. The effects of thermocoagulation were studied in vitro in fresh egg whites, using time intervals of 20, 40, 60, 80 and 100 s, and in vivo, in the subcortical white matter of 20 adult New Zealand white rabbits. Animals were sacrificed after 7 days. Lesions were photographed and measured under magnification. In all cases, the coagulated masses were ellipsoid, with regular, well-demarcated borders. A two-way statistical analysis of variance was done. The coagulum size increased with higher temperatures and with larger probes. The increase was significant in both diameter and length ($p = 0.001$). In contrast, the use of different times at the same level of temperature showed no significant increase in most of the electrodes. There were two statistical significant time effects, for both diameter and length, with the monopolar 2-mm electrode. The use of real-time monitoring with graphic display and the feedback information provided for the computerized control of power and current allows high precision of the temperature at the electrode tip during the production of the lesion.

1011–6125/92/0584–0121 $ 2.75/0

Introduction

For many years radiofrequency-generated lesions have been used for different purposes, including the treatment of pain or abnormal movements [1]. More sophisticated equipment is continuously being developed in an attempt to improve the precision of the size of the lesion. However, the reliability of this method has been questioned because of the variation in the size of lesions produced by the electrode at different times and temperatures [2].

The purpose of the present study was to determine the size of the lesion produced by different electrodes and a radiofrequency generator provided with a computerized feedback mechanism that keeps the electrode tip temperature constant during lesion production, regardless of varying tissue impedence. Eight electrodes of different size and tip characteristics were evaluated at different temperatures and time settings, both in vitro and in vivo.

The accuracy of this computerized control was evaluated, as well as the reliability of lesions produced by each electrode.

Materials and Methods

A 500-kHz radiofrequency generator (Fischer, Freiburg, FRG) provided with a computerized program and a microchip in the head of the electrodes allowed recording and monitoring of stimulation, temperature, time and impedance parameters on the electrode tip (fig. 1). This information was fed into the computerized generator and used as feedback information to control voltage and current. The final goal was to produce a lesion at a desired constant temperature.

The electrodes were monopolar 1 mm (tips 1.5 and 3 mm length), monopolar 2 mm (tip 4 mm length), bipolar 1 mm (tip 4.5 mm length), bipolar 2 mm (tip 6 mm length), bipolar asymmetric 1 mm (tip 3 mm length) and bipolar string (tips 1.5 and 3 mm length fig. 2). Continuous graphic display of voltage, current, impedance and temperature was obtained using an interfaced printer. For visual documentation of the lesion, a Minolta camera (×370), adapted to a Zeiss OPMI 1 microscope, was used. The dimensions considered were the maximum diamter and length of the lesions. The mean and SD of the lesions were calculated and tabulated. Statistical analysis was performed using a two-way analysis of variance (ANOVA).

In vitro Studies

The effects of radiofrequency current were studied in a hen's fresh egg white, warmed to 37 °C. Egg white was chosen because of its protein content and coagulation properties and because its translucency allows easy visualization of the lesions either directly or by photography. The egg white was placed in a round glass container. Probes

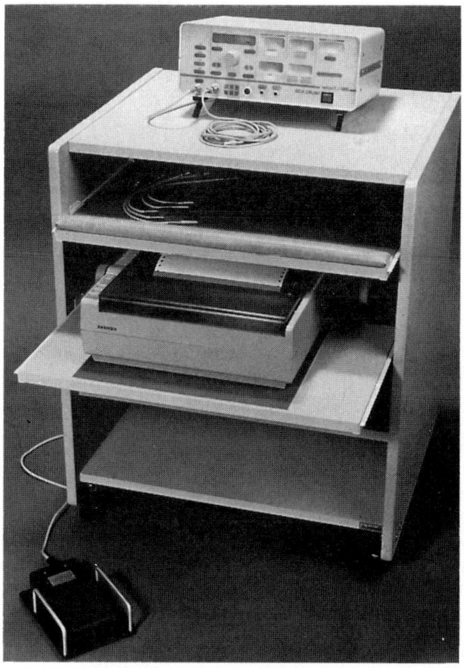

Fig. 1. Radiofrequency generator Neuro N 50 (Fischer, Freiburg, FRG).

were secured with a micromanipulator and advanced carefully until the tips were completely immersed. For monopolar coagulation, the ground electrode (reference electrode) was a thin metal plate pressed against the inner side of the wall of the glass container. Coagulation was successively produced at different temperatures (65, 70, 75, 80, 85 and 90 °C) and at different times (20, 40, 60, 80 and 100 s). Each lesion was repeated 5 times, for a total of 150 lesions for each electrode (i.e. a total of 1,200 lesions). Lesions were observed under the microscope and photographed with a 1-mm scaled plate under the lesion. Final measurement of the lesions was obtained using the photographs with magnification.

In vivo Studies

To determine the effects in vivo, 4 electrodes (bipolar 1 mm, tip 4.5 mm; bipolar 2 mm, tip 6 mm; monopolar 1 mm, tip 3 mm; monopolar 2 mm, tip 4 mm) were evaluated in the subcortical white matter of 20 adult New Zealand white rabbits. The rats were anesthetized with intravenous pentobarbital (30 mg/kg), and placed in a Kopf stereotactic frame. A midline incision was made on the scalp to expose the sagittal suture. Using a high-speed drill, a frontoparietal 3-mm craniectomy was performed on the left side, 1–2 mm anterior to the coronal suture and 5 mm lateral to the sagittal suture. The

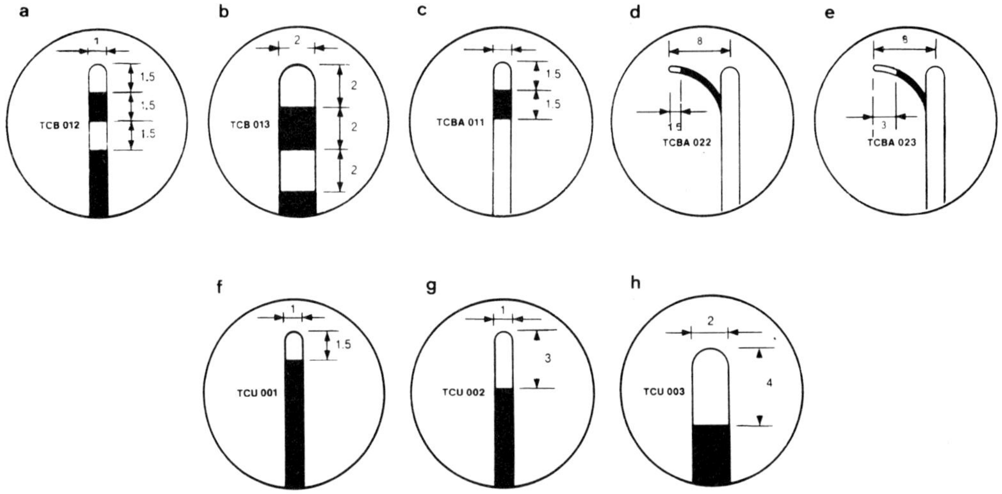

Fig. 2. Different electrodes used. **a** Bipolar, 1 mm diameter (tip length 4.5 mm). **b** Bipolar, 2 mm diameter (tip 6 mm length). **c** Bipolar asymmetric, 1 mm diameter (tip 3 mm length). **d** Bipolar string (tip 1.5 mm length). **e** Bipolar string (tip 3 mm length). **f** Monopolar, 1 mm diameter (tip 1.5 mm length). **g** Bipolar, 1 mm diameter (tip 3 mm length). **h** Monopolar, 2 mm diameter (tip 4 mm length).

dura was opened with a linear incision, and the tip of the probe was advanced with a microdrive through the cortical layer, to a depth of 8 mm. The electrodes were randomyl assigned and the lesions were produced using 80 °C during 60 s in all cases. After the coagulation, the temperature curve drop was followed, and the probe was removed after 40 °C had been reached. Animals were killed 7 days after the procedure by an intravenous overdose of pentobarbital, and the brains were fixed by intraarterial injection of 5% formalin solution and removed. They were immersed in 5% formalin solution for 1 week. Then blocks of the tissue were embedded in paraffin, sectioned in slices and stained with hematoxylin and eosin. The slides were observed under a microscope and measured with a graded scale.

Results

In vitro reproducible, well-formed lesions were obtained. The coagulum developed as an ovoid opacification of the egg white and originated in both ends of the exposed electrode tip. Its borders were always regular and well demarcated (fig. 3).

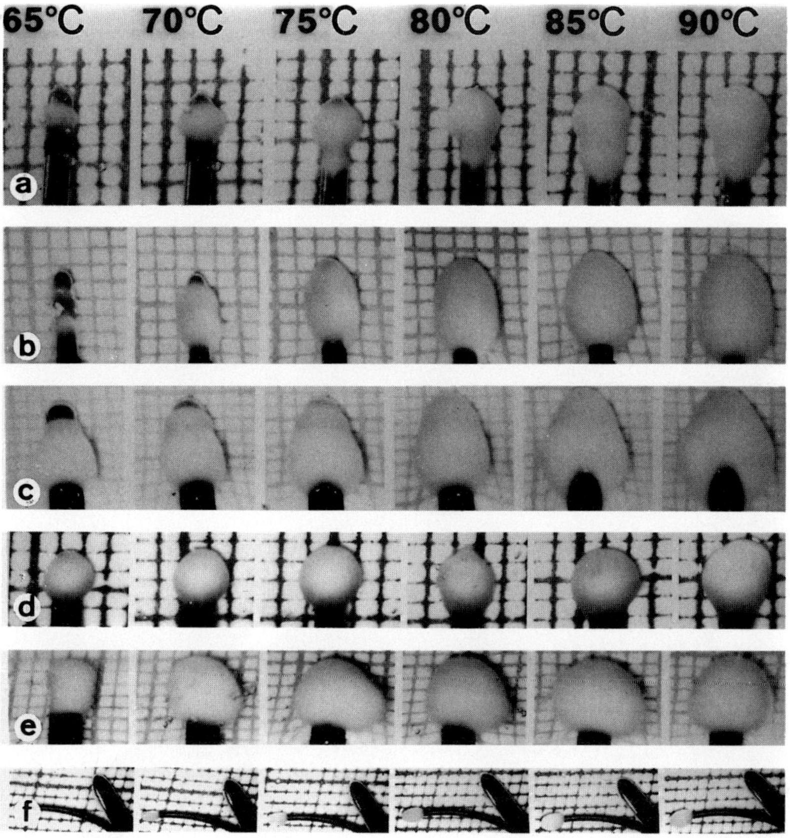

Fig. 3. Lesions obtained with different electrodes at different temperatures. **a** Bipolar asymmetric, 1 mm diameter. **b** Bipolar, 1 mm diameter. **c** Bipolar, 2 mm diameter. **d** Monopolar, 1 mm diameter. **e** monopolar, 2 mm diameter. **f** Bipolar string (tip 1.5 mm).

On histological sections, the lesions produced in the brains of the rabbits were ellipsoid, with a central area of coagulation necrosis and cellular proliferation, predominantly macrophages, on the periphery. In some cases, a vascular proliferation was found around the lesion (fig. 4). Signs of boiling or carbonization were not present in any lesion. During the production of the lesion, the temperature graphic described a smoothly ascending curve from 37 °C to the desired level of temperature (65, 70, 75, 80, 85, 90 °C), followed by a straight horizontal

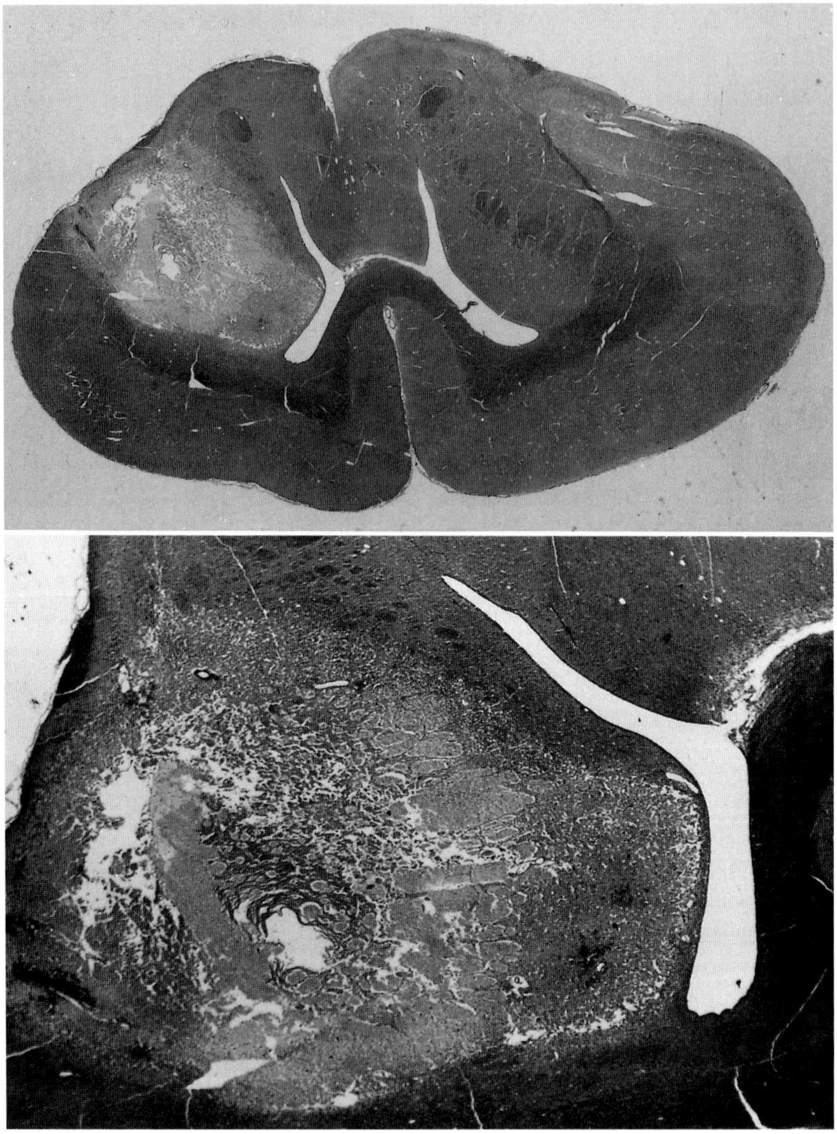

a

b

Fig. 4. Morphological aspect of a coagulation lesion in the subcortical structures of a rabbit, 7 days after the production of the lesion. Parameters were electrode bipolar, 1 mm diameter (4 mm tip); temperature, 80 °C; time, 60 s. Stained with hematoxylin and eosin. **a** × 8.2. **b** × 17.6.

Table 1. Diameter (D) and length (L) of lesions produced by electrode of 1 mm diameter with tip of 4.5 mm length

Time s	Temperature, °C											
	65		70		75		80		85		90	
	D	L	D	L	D	L	D	L	D	L	D	L
20	–	–	1.91 ±0.1	2.95 ±0.4	2.12 ±0.1	3.64 ±0.74	2.36 ±0.2	4.40 ±0.78	2.67 ±0.3	4.63 ±0.86	2.76 ±0.27	4.78 ±0.56
40	–	–	1.98 ±0.04	3.00 ±0.45	2.37 ±0.32	3.85 ±0.80	2.36 ±0.27	4.72 ±0.68	2.77 ±0.5	4.82 ±0.58	2.77 ±0.3	4.96 ±0.64
60	–	–	2.20 ±0.4	3.06 ±0.46	2.42 ±0.07	3.85 ±0.80	2.54 ±0.26	4.74 ±0.70	3.16 ±0.6	4.96 ±0.50	2.86 ±0.4	5.05 ±0.43
80	1.00 ±0.0	2.40 ±0.37	2.12 ±0.2	3.27 ±0.66	2.42 ±0.07	3.95 ±0.68	2.72 ±0.4	4.79 ±0.63	2.98 ±0.47	4.88 ±0.61	2.90 ±0.5	5.13 ±0.47
100	1.99 ±0.1	2.60 ±0.37	2.16 ±0.12	3.62 ±0.7	2.34 ±0.18	3.95 ±0.64	2.66 ±0.47	4.82 ±0.60	2.93 ±0.5	4.93 ±0.65	3.10 ±0.6	5.21 ±0.54

line at this predetermined level. The corresponding curves of voltage (volts), radiofrequency current (amperes) and power (watts) showed in initial increase and were maintained in a plateau line with small oscillations.

The mean and SD of diameter and length of all lesions produced in vitro are shown in tables 1–8. Table 9 shows the results of the lesions produced in vivo.

Two-way ANOVA allowed us to examine the data obtained in vitro for time effects, degree effects and type of electrode. The coagulum size increased with higher temperatures and with larger probe size. The increase was significant in both diameter and length of the lesion ($p = 0.001$). The use of different times at the same level of temperature showed no significant increase in size for most of the electrodes (from 20 up to 100 s). There were only two statistically significant time effects for both length and diameter with the monopolar 2-mm electrode (table 8). However, with other electrodes, measurements showed a slight increase in size, although they were not statistically significant (tables 1–7).

Table 2. Diameter (D) and length (L) of lesions produced by bipolar asymmetric electrode of 1 mm diameter with tip of 3 mm length

Time s	Temperature, °C											
	65		70		75		80		85		90	
	D	L	D	L	D	L	D	L	D	L	D	L
20	1.70 ±0.19	1.65 ±0.20	2.18 ±0.22	2.10 ±0.34	2.45 ±0.10	2.85 ±0.12	2.80 ±0.19	3.30 ±0.24	2.93 ±0.29	3.80 ±0.19	3.10 ±0.34	4.10 ±0.12
40	1.80 ±0.19	1.72 ±0.17	2.20 ±0.24	2.15 ±0.30	2.55 ±0.29	2.90 ±0.12	2.91 ±0.25	3.50 ±0.16	3.00 ±0.27	4.00 ±0.00	3.10 ±0.34	4.20 ±0.24
60	1.85 ±0.12	1.85 ±0.34	2.25 ±0.32	2.25 ±0.22	2.57 ±0.29	3.00 ±0.00	3.03 ±0.34	3.55 ±0.10	3.05 ±0.37	4.10 ±0.20	3.10 ±0.34	4.20 ±0.24
80	1.88 ±0.11	1.85 ±0.34	2.25 ±0.32	2.25 ±0.22	2.62 ±0.32	3.00 ±0.00	3.00 ±0.32	3.60 ±0.12	3.15 ±0.46	4.10 ±0.20	3.16 ±0.33	4.30 ±0.24
100	1.88 ±0.11	1.85 ±0.34	2.25 ±0.32	2.30 ±0.29	2.64 ±0.34	3.00 ±0.00	3.10 ±0.37	3.60 ±0.12	3.25 ±0.47	4.10 ±0.20	3.31 ±0.47	4.30 ±0.24

Table 3. Diameter (D) and length (L) of lesions produced by bipolar electrode of 2 mm diameter with tip of 6 mm length

Time s	Temperature, °C											
	65		70		75		80		85		90	
	D	L	D	L	D	L	D	L	D	L	D	L
20	3.65 ±0.7	3.30 ±0.7	3.90 ±0.1	4.00 ±1.1	3.90 ±0.2	4.64 ±0.47	4.40 ±0.4	5.30 ±1.68	4.70 ±0.7	5.40 ±1.9	4.20 ±0.5	4.46 ±0.5
40	3.70 ±0.4	3.50 ±0.6	3.90 ±0.20	4.60 ±0.9	4.30 ±0.5	4.82 ±1.52	4.50 ±0.44	5.56 ±1.9	4.50 ±0.8	5.14 ±1.8	4.00 ±0.42	5.30 ±0.8
60	4.00 ±0.2	3.90 ±1.1	4.10 ±0.4	4.40 ±1.4	4.60 ±0.5	4.86 ±1.56	4.50 ±0.6	5.46 ±1.9	4.50 ±0.67	4.74 ±1.7	4.30 ±0.20	5.30 ±0.8
80	4.00 ±0.3	3.94 ±1.1	4.10 ±0.4	4.46 ±1.4	4.60 ±0.47	5.22 ±1.7	4.60 ±0.66	5.34 ±2.0	4.90 ±0.74	4.90 ±1.8	4.00 ±0.66	5.40 ±1.0
100	4.10 ±0.3	4.00 ±1.2	4.10 ±0.4	4.54 ±1.4	4.80 ±0.25	4.68 ±1.8	4.80 ±0.64	5.62 ±1.9	5.00 ±0.90	4.98 ±1.5	4.20 ±0.80	4.96 ±0.9

Table 4. Diameter (D) and length (L) of lesions produced by bipolar string with tip of 5 mm length

Time s	Temperature, °C											
	65		70		75		80		85		90	
	D	L	D	L	D	L	D	L	D	L	D	L
20	1.00 ±0.00	1.35 ±0.12	1.04 ±0.08	1.50 ±0.00	1.33 ±0.19	1.85 ±0.20	1.66 ±0.26	1.95 ±0.10	1.75 ±0.22	2.00 ±0.00	1.93 ±0.25	2.28 ±0.06
40	1.00 ±0.00	1.35 ±0.12	1.25 ±0.16	1.56 ±0.05	1.40 ±0.12	1.85 ±0.20	1.66 ±0.26	2.00 ±0.00	1.80 ±0.28	2.05 ±0.10	2.01 ±0.22	2.38 ±0.11
60	1.00 ±0.00	1.35 ±0.12	1.25 ±0.16	1.62 ±0.11	1.40 ±0.12	1.85 ±0.20	1.70 ±0.29	2.00 ±0.00	1.86 ±0.34	2.10 ±0.12	2.06 ±0.24	2.40 ±0.12
80	1.00 ±0.00	1.35 ±0.12	1.30 ±0.10	1.62 ±0.11	1.40 ±0.12	1.85 ±0.20	1.75 ±0.32	2.00 ±0.00	1.88 ±0.34	2.10 ±0.12	2.08 ±0.22	2.40 ±0.12
100	1.00 ±0.00	1.40 ±0.12	1.30 ±0.10	1.65 ±0.12	1.44 ±0.16	1.85 ±0.20	1.75 ±0.32	2.00 ±0.00	1.93 ±0.37	2.15 ±0.12	2.08 ±0.22	2.45 ±0.19

Table 5. Diameter (D) and length (L) of lesions produced by bipolar string with tip of 3 mm length

Time s	Temperature, °C											
	65		70		75		80		85		90	
	D	L	D	L	D	L	D	L	D	L	D	L
20	1.28 ±0.23	2.50 ±0.70	1.47 ±0.34	2.34 ±0.42	1.79 ±0.36	2.66 ±0.33	1.75 ±0.41	2.72 ±0.34	2.01 ±0.38	2.62 ±0.47	2.06 ±0.57	3.04 ±0.48
40	1.34 ±0.31	2.24 ±0.7	1.54 ±0.26	2.54 ±0.45	1.80 ±0.42	2.66 ±0.33	1.73 ±0.41	2.74 ±0.29	2.07 ±0.31	2.72 ±0.58	2.24 ±0.69	3.12 ±0.55
60	1.36 ±0.37	2.22 ±0.6	1.56 ±0.29	2.70 ±0.40	1.79 ±0.39	2.70 ±0.38	1.86 ±0.36	2.64 ±0.27	2.08 ±0.33	2.76 ±0.5	2.26 ±0.67	2.96 ±0.3
80	1.36 ±0.37	2.50 ±0.5	1.46 ±0.33	2.72 ±0.41	1.88 ±0.51	2.72 ±0.36	1.99 ±0.45	2.90 ±0.26	2.11 ±0.37	2.78 ±0.5	2.34 ±0.62	2.94 ±0.3
100	1.44 ±0.39	2.50 ±0.5	1.78 ±0.26	2.70 ±0.4	1.92 ±0.52	2.74 ±0.37	1.99 ±0.43	3.06 ±0.42	2.24 ±0.50	3.00 ±0.47	2.38 ±0.63	3.00 ±0.42

Table 6. Diameter (D) and length (L) of lesions produced by monopolar electrode of 1 mm diameter with tip of 5 mm length

Time s	Temperature, °C											
	65		70		75		80		85		90	
	D	L	D	L	D	L	D	L	D	L	D	L
20	2.01	2.18	2.25	2.75	2.45	3.00	2.75	3.48	3.05	3.90	3.22	4.15
	±0.22	±0.22	±0.23	±0.16	±0.20	±0.00	±0.50	±0.24	±0.37	±0.20	±0.39	±0.20
40	2.10	2.20	2.33	2.76	2.60	3.05	2.82	3.55	1.13	4.00	3.32	4.30
	±0.20	±0.24	±0.25	±0.16	±0.34	±0.10	±0.47	±0.24	±0.44	±0.24	±0.47	±0.19
60	2.10	2.20	2.33	2.83	2.70	3.25	2.90	3.55	3.18	4.05	3.39	4.30
	±0.20	±0.24	±0.25	±0.10	±0.4	±0.16	±0.45	±0.24	±0.41	±0.10	±0.56	±0.19
80	2.10	2.25	2.45	2.90	2.70	3.40	2.98	3.70	3.25	4.15	3.39	4.45
	±0.20	±0.22	±0.29	±0.12	±0.4	±0.12	±0.46	±0.37	±0.5	±0.12	±0.50	±0.19
100	2.10	2.30	2.45	2.95	2.70	3.40	3.05	3.80	3.25	4.25	3.39	4.65
	±0.20	±0.24	±0.20	±0.10	±0.4	±0.12	±0.48	±0.43	±0.50	±0.22	±0.50	±0.20

Table 7. Diameter (D) and length (L) of lesions produced by monopolar electrode of 1 mm diameter with tip of 3 mm length

Time s	Temperature, °C											
	65		70		75		80		85		90	
	D	L	D	L	D	L	D	L	D	L	D	L
20	1.98	1.70	2.40	2.50	2.62	3.00	3.26	3.80	3.40	4.06	4.26	4.36
	±0.25	±0.5	±0.20	±0.50	±0.22	±0.7	±0.43	±0.5	±0.69	±0.6	±0.80	±0.72
40	2.09	1.70	2.49	2.73	2.87	3.30	3.03	3.84	3.89	4.18	4.58	4.36
	±0.24	±0.4	±0.18	±0.8	±0.23	±0.5	±0.40	±0.6	±0.80	±0.74	±0.80	±0.7
60	2.15	2.10	2.53	2.79	3.01	3.48	3.38	3.88	4.07	4.16	4.80	4.44
	±0.25	±0.57	±0.25	±0.9	±0.26	±0.6	±0.6	±0.6	±0.8	±0.70	±1.2	±0.88
80	2.24	2.14	2.57	2.69	3.16	3.46	3.55	3.92	4.16	4.40	4.46	4.80
	±0.25	±0.59	±0.24	±0.9	±0.28	±0.67	±0.7	±0.67	±0.18	±0.79	±0.7	±0.68
100	2.20	2.14	2.57	2.65	3.17	3.51	3.77	4.08	4.21	4.40	4.63	4.90
	±0.26	±0.6	±0.18	±0.9	±0.30	±0.6	±0.75	±0.73	±0.7	±0.65	±0.66	±0.54

Table 8. Diameter (D) and length (L) of lesions produced by monopolar electrode of 2 mm diameter with tip of 4 mm length

Time s	Temperature, °C											
	65		70		75		80		85		90	
	D	L	D	L	D	L	D	L	D	L	D	L
20	3.40 ±0.5	3.38 ±1.00	3.75 ±0.28	4.60 ±0.4	4.56 ±0.28	4.56 ±0.7	5.00 ±0.27	5.09 ±0.6	5.45 ±0.55	5.44 ±0.8	5.68 ±1.00	6.29 ±0.45
40	3.46 ±0.5	3.90 ±0.5	4.16 ±0.13	4.80 ±0.56	4.76 ±0.59	4.86 ±0.67	5.00 ±0.57	5.16 ±0.50	5.55 ±0.50	5.72 ±0.60	5.98 ±1.00	6.19 ±0.50
60	3.76 ±0.6	4.24 ±0.58	4.15 ±0.14	4.74 ±0.57	4.66 ±0.41	4.90 ±0.6	5.26 ±0.50	5.30 ±0.6	5.69 ±0.69	5.78 ±0.57	6.17 ±1.00	6.55 ±0.55
80	3.65 ±0.43	4.00 ±0.47	4.41 ±0.48	4.90 ±0.54	4.98 ±0.63	4.80 ±0.56	5.38 ±0.46	5.58 ±0.6	5.58 ±0.80	5.98 ±0.58	6.03 ±0.90	6.49 ±0.67
100	3.82 ±0.57	4.24 ±0.48	4.60 ±0.37	4.98 ±0.50	5.16 ±0.49	5.06 ±0.37	5.68 ±0.7	5.68 ±0.64	5.93 ±0.7	6.30 ±0.45	6.23 ±0.8	6.63 ±0.48

Table 9. Size of lesions in vivo (80 °C, 60 s)

Electrode	Lesion	
	diameter	lenght
Bipolar 1 mm (tip 4.5 mm)	4.20 ± 0.24	5.75 ± 0.22
Bipolar 2 mm (tip 6 mm)	5.25 ± 0.38	6.06 ± 0.33
Monopolar 1 mm (tip 4 mm)	4.91 ± 0.41	6.22 ± 0.20
Monopolar 2 mm (tip 4 mm)	5.5 ± 0.17	7.36 ± 0.25

The comparison between monopolar and bipolar electrodes (ANOVA) showed a significant difference. In the case of 2-mm electrodes, the monopolar produced larger lesions in both diameter and length. With 1-mm electrodes, the monopolar device produced larger-diameter but smaller-length, lesions than the bipolar.

Discussion

Among the various methods to produce lesions in the central nervous system, radiofrequency thermocoagulation has gained widespread acceptance in functional and stereotactic neurosurgery [3–5]. Important factors determine the size of the lesion: the temperature, electrode configuration (monopolar or bipolar) and characteristic of the tissues [3, 4, 6]. Previous reports have demonstrated the importance of temperature monitoring for the reliability and predictability of the lesion size [3, 4, 6, 7]. Reversible lesions have been produced in cats using temperatures between 40 and 49 °C [8]. Clinically, temperatures between 70 and 80 °C have been recomended [9] for the production of irreversible thermocontrolled lesions. Although the lesion size increases with higher temperatures, the risk of producing boiling or carbonization of tissues also increases. Lower temperatures may produce reversible lesions with the corresponding recurrence of the symptoms. Because the time of application at constant temperature is less critical in determining the lesion's size, the use of long times is therefore not recommended. Another factor influencing the size of the lesion is the use of monopolar versus bipolar electrodes [3, 6, 10]. In our study, the lesion produced by monopolar electrodes continues to increase as the temperature increases; for the bipolar device, there appears to be a threshold at which the size no longer continues to increase (85 °C and higher). The findings in vivo were slightly different from those in vitro; however the lesion was slightly larger. In all cases, the lesions were reliable and predictable, as shown by the small SDs. We believe it is advisable for the neurosurgeon to keep these tables as a reference parameter during the intraoperative produre. In vitro lesions represent an adequate model for the study of the physical characteristics of lesions produced by radiofrequency. Real-time monitoring with graphic display provides an adequate control of the physical parameters.

We feel that the addition of the feedback mechanism for the computerized control of power and current allowed for higher precision of the temperature at the electrode tip during the production of the lesion, i.e. the temperature was kept constant during the present time. A priori knowledge of the expected size of lesions is an important factor for the optimization of functional procedures.

References

1 Fager CA: Surgical treatment of involuntary movement disorders. Lahey Clin Found Bull 1973;22:79–83.
2 Sweet WH, Mark VH, Hamlin H: Radiofrequency lesions in the central nervous system of man and cat. J Neurosurg 1960;17:213–225.
3 Alberts WW, Wright EW Jr, Feinstein B, von Bonin G: Experimental radiofrequency brain lesion size as a function of physical parameters. J Neurosurg 1966; 25:421–423.
4 Bonin GV, Alberts WW, Wright EW Jr, et al: Radiofrequency brain lesions: Size as function of physical parameters. Arch Neurol (Chicago) 1965;12:25–29.
5 Cosman ER, Cosman BJ: Methods of making nervous system lesions; in Wilkins RH, Rengachary SS (eds): Neurosurgery. New York, McGraw-Hill, 1984.
6 Diekmann G, Gabriel E, Hassler R: Size, form and structural peculiarities of experimental brain lesions obtained by thermocontrolled radiofrequency. Confin Neurol 1965;26:134–142.
7 Cosman ER, Nashold BS, Bedenbaugh P: Stereotactic radiofrequency lesion making. Appl Neurophysiol 1983;46:160–166.
8 Brodkey JS, Miyazaki Y, Ervin FR, Mark VH: Reversible heat lesions with radiofrequency current: A method of stereotactic localization. J Neurosurg 1964;21: 49–53.
9 Moringlane JR, Koch R, Schafer H, Ostertag ChB: Experimental radiofrequency coagulation with computer-based on-line monitoring of temperature and power. Acta Neurochir 1989;96:126–131.
10 Organ LW: Electrophysiologic principles of radiofrequency lesion making. Appl Neurophysiol 1976;39:69–76.

Lucia Zamorano, University Health Center, Department of Neurosurgery, 4201 St. Antoine UHC/6E, Detroit, MI 48201 (USA)

Proceedings of the Meeting of the American Society for Stereotactic and Functional Neurosurgery, Pittsburgh, Pa., June 16–19, 1991
Stereotact Funct Neurosurg 1992;58:134–140

Positron Emission Tomography Imaging-Directed Stereotactic Neurosurgery

Robert J. Maciunas, Robert M. Kessler, Calvin Maurer, Venkat Mandava, Graham Watt, Gregory Smith

Departments of Neurological Surgery, Diagnostic Radiology, Computer Science and Biomedical Engineering, Vanderbilt University Medical Center, Nashville, Tenn., USA

Key Words. Positron emission tomography · PET · FDG · Fluorodeoxyglucose · Stereotaxy · Biopsy · Glioma · Imaging · Tumor

Abstract. The diagnostic yield of stereotactic biopsies depends upon safely sampling the most representative regions of masses. Potentially, localization information presently available from CT and MR scans might be improved by considering regional levels of cerebral metabolism by PET. In 10 selected stereotactic biopsies of intracranial mass lesions, PET scans were obtained using the Siemens CTI system; the Kelly-Goerss Compass system was used as the stereotactic development platform. PET-[^{18}F]-fluorodeoxyglucose (FDG) images provided clinically significant information by appropriately directing biopsy efforts when CT and MRI was inconclusive or misleading. PET-FDG images can be successfully incorporated into routine image-directed stereotactic surgery.

Image-directed stereotactic biopsy provides a high percentage of correct histopathologic diagnoses of intracranial mass lesions. The diagnostic yield of stereotatic biopsies depends upon safely sampling the most representative regions of masses. Various strategies have been described for best interpreting preoperative imaging studies to select the most diagnostic region(s) for biopsy. Localization information presently available from CT and MR scans, although excellent, is not infallible. Potentially, localization might be improved by considering regional levels of cerebral metabolism data that are unique to PET. PET data depicting fluorine-18-fluorodeoxy-*D*-glucose ([^{18}F]-FDG) uptake have previously been shown to provide a functional diagnosis of

1011–6125/92/0584–0134 $ 2.75/0

tumor activity, but with limited spatial resolution. To overcome this limitation, we (1) instituted a protocol for obtaining high-resolution cranial PET-FDG images, and (2) developed stereotactic instrumentation and surgical treatment planning software to spatially correlate CT-, MR-, DSA- and PET-derived imaging sets. PET scans were obtained using the Siemens CTI system; the Kelly-Goerss Compass system was used as the stereotactic development platform.

Methods

Data Acquisition

The Kelly-Goerss Compass stereotactic frame was applied in the usual fashion. The carbon fiber pins are inserted into 4 holes drilled through the outer table of the skull into the diploe. The carbon fiber fixation system allowed frame reapplication following data acquisition when indicated by reference to recorded micrometer settings on the fixation pins.

A Siemens DR-H CT scanner was used to obtain contrast-enhanced stereotactic CT scan data sets. Four-millimeter-thick slices were routinely employed. A Siemens Magnetom 1.5-tesla coil magnet MRI scanner was used to obtain a series of stereotactic MR images. A standard data set was made up of axial T_1-weighted, proton density, T_2-weighted and gadolinium-enhanced T_1-weighted images. Other sequences were obtained as clinically indicated.

A standard N-bar fiducial localization system is employed by the Compass stereotactic device for registration of scan images to the head frame. The localization fiducials are made of carbon fiber for CT imaging, and are hollow tubes filled with dilute gadolinium/water solution for the MRI.

Positron Emission Tomography

PET was performed with a Siemens CTI model positron tomograph, which has 3,072 BGO detectors arranged in 8 circular rings around a 54-cm-diameter opening. The axial field of view is 12.0 cm. In-plane resolution is approximately 6 mm, while axial resolution is 8 mm. The resulting image set is composed of fifteen 128 × 128 matrix contiguous slices with a pixel size of 2.5 × 2.5 mm and a slice thickness of 8 mm. The image matrix is interpolated to a 256 × 256 matrix for display purposes by the intraoperative stereotactic image-processing computer.

Transmission images were obtained to correct for photon attenuation. Emission images were obtained 35 min after intravenous injection of 10 μCi of FDG. The transmission images were obtained with the stereotactic N-bar localizing fiducial system in place and filled with water.

Emission images were obtained in 15 planes for 17 min. The emission images were obtained after filling the stereotactic N-bar localizing fiducial system with 5 μCi/ml of FDG solution. After considerable phantom testing with putative contrast agents for the localization fiducial system, this was found to be superior in producing excellent visualization of the fiducials while not exceeding the maximum intensity in the brain. This factor was critical in maintaining a good dynamic range and signal-to-noise ratio for the brain parenchyma in these stereotactic image sets.

During image acquisition, blood samples were periodically drawn from a venous access port from the hand contralateral to the site of FDG injection. Radioactivity and plasma glucose concentration were assayed to convert tissue FDG radioactivity into glucose metabolic rate. For this conversion, the standard Sokoloff model and the kinetic constants for FDG as determined by Phelp et al. were used.

Stereotactic Image Processing and Surgical Treatment Planning

The scan images are stored on 9-in magnetic tape for transport to the intraoperative stereotatic image-processing computer. A Sun SPARCserver 4-400 is used as the host computer at our institution, networked to a Sun 3-160/Vicom VME unit. Once the images are loaded onto the image memory of the intraoperative computer, the neurosurgeon reviews the correlated images. Target selection is accomplished by reference to a simultaneous onscreen display of the correlated CT, T_2-weighted MRI, T_1-weighted MRI with gadolinium, T_1-weighted MRI without gadolinium, and the PET scans. Target selection in any imaging screen is automatically correlated in real time with simultaneously displayed cursors on all the other imaging modalities. Once the appropriate target point and entry point have been tentatively selected on the correlated images, interactive trajectory planning is carried out using a multimodality multiplanar display array.

Results and Conclusion

In 10 selected stereotactic biopsies of intracranial mass lesions, the addition of PET-FDG imaging provided critical localization information when CT and MRI was inconclusive or misleading (fig. 1, 2). In 2 cases of Daumas-DuPort type 3 gliomas comprised of infiltrating tumor cells, PET-FDG appropriately directed the biopsy to regions of maximally aggressive tumor. In these cases, the diagnosis was revised from astrocytoma to anaplastic astrocytoma. In 1 patient with a low-grade fibrillary infiltrating astrocytoma, the PET scan suggested a region of slightly increased metabolism within a field of sharply diminished metabolism. This region demonstrated a significantly greater degree of infiltrating tumor cells than other more hypometabolic regions nearby, which were better visualized on CT and T_2-weighted MRI. In 1

Fig. 1. a Correlated CT, T_2-MRI, T_1-Gd-MRI, PD-MRI and PET, demonstrating hypermetabolism in the solid tumor tissue of a glioblastoma. **b** Hypometabolism within the region of infiltrating tumor cells of a glioblastoma.

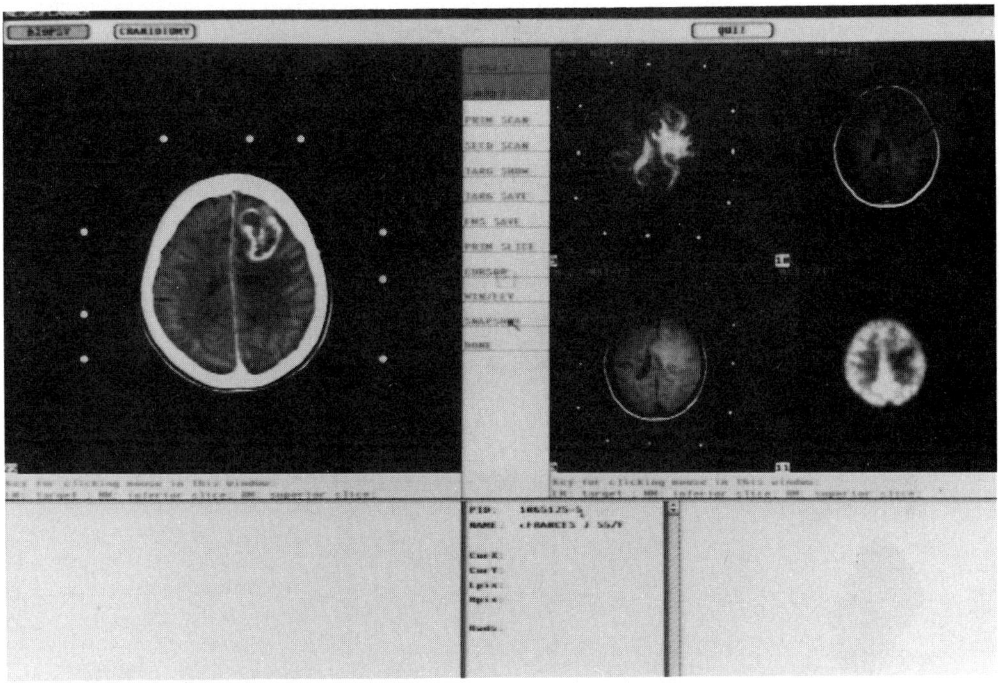
BIOPSY
CRANIOTOMY
QUIT
PRIM SCAN
SEED SCAN
TARG SHOW
TARG SAVE
FMS SAVE
PRIM SLICE
CURSOR
WIN/LEV
SNAPSHOT
DONE
Key for clicking mouse in this window:
LM: target ; MM: inferior slice; RM: superior slice.

1a

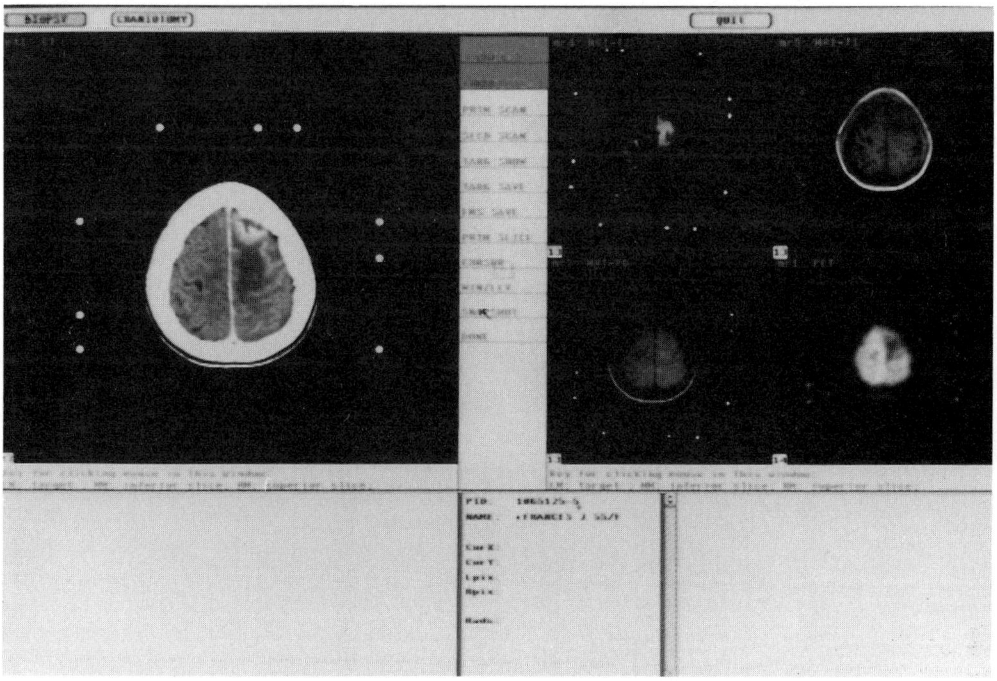
BIOPSY
CRANIOTOMY
QUIT
PRIM SCAN
SEED SCAN
TARG SHOW
TARG SAVE
FMS SAVE
PRIM SLICE
CURSOR
WIN/LEV
DONE
Key for clicking mouse in this window:
LM: target ; MM: inferior slice; RM: superior slice.

1b

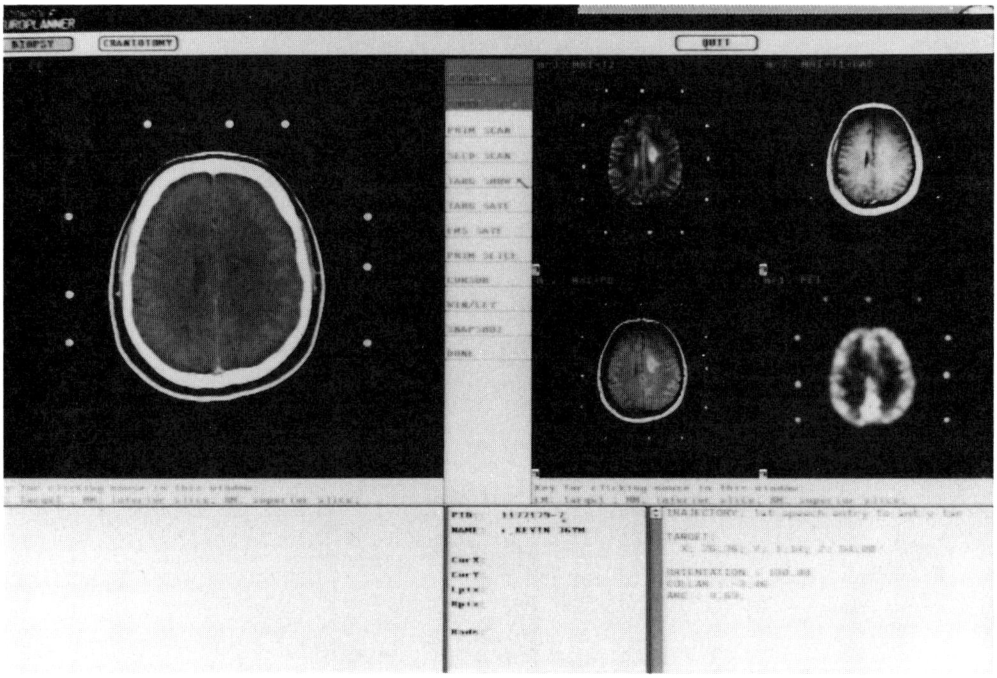
BIOPSY
CRANIOTOMY
QUIT
PRIM SCAN
SECD SCAN
CURSOR
WIN/LEV
DONE
PID:
NAME:
CurX:
CurY:
Lptx:
Rptx:
Rads:
TARGET:

2a

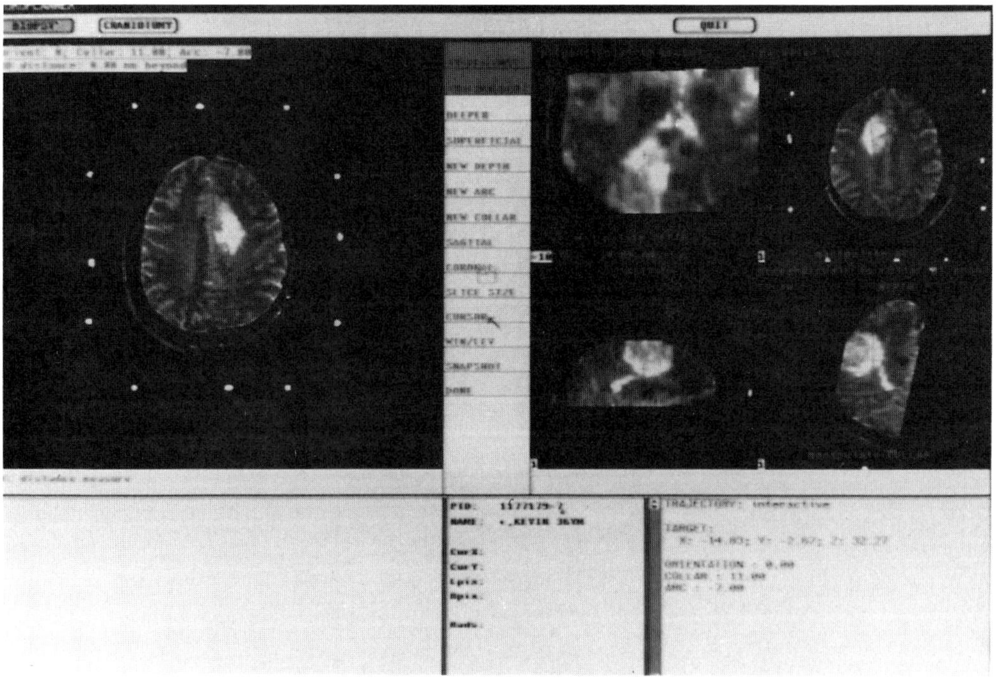
BIOPSY
CRANIOTOMY
QUIT
DEEPER
SUPERFICIAL
NEW DEPTH
NEW ARC
NEW COLLAR
SAGITAL
SLICE SIZE
CURSOR
WIN/LEV
SNAPSHOT
DONE
PID:
NAME:
CurX:
CurY:
Lptx:
Rptx:
Rads:
TRAJECTORY: interactive
TARGET:

2b

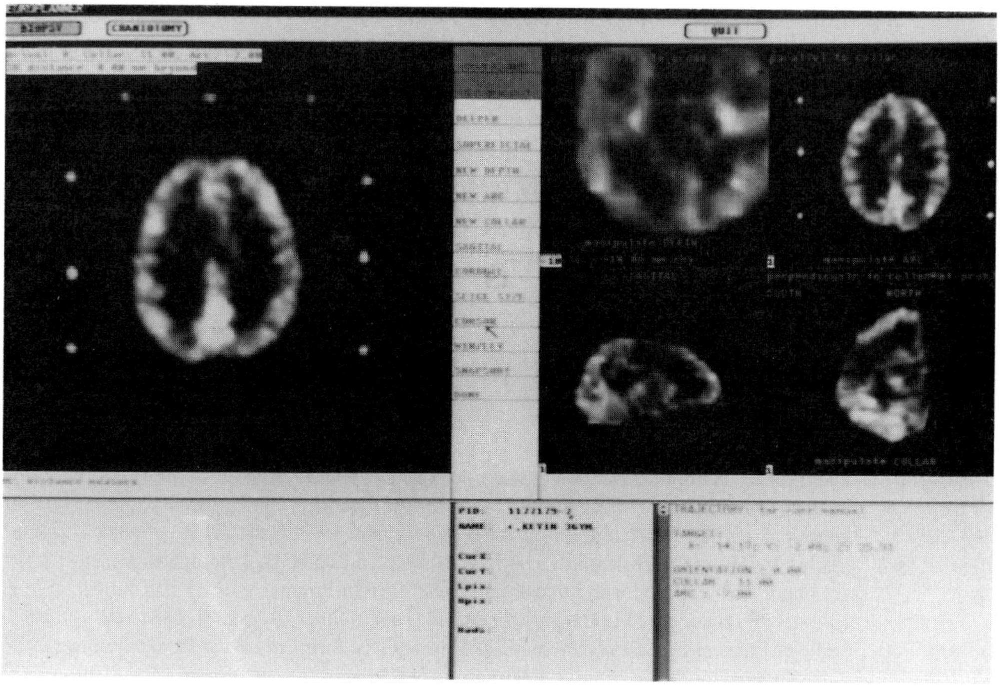

2c

Fig. 2. a Correlated CT, T_2-MRI, T_1-Gd-MRI, PD-MRI and PET demonstrating a focal periventricular hypermetabolic region of anaplastic astrocytoma within what otherwise appeared to be a low-grade infiltrative astrocytoma. **b** Interactive planning of biopsy using T_2-MR images. **c** Interactive planning of biopsy using PET images.

patient with a normal CT, a hypometabolic region correlated with a small bright region on T_2-weighted MRI, which proved to be an infiltrating low-grade astrocytoma. In 2 cases, PET demonstrated focal hypermetabolic regions that proved to be small nodules of recurrent glioblastoma multiform solid tumor tissue within larger regions of postradiation changes. The clinical course of these patients has been more consistent with that of recurrent glioblastoma. Focal hypermetabolism within a ring-enhancing glioma on CT and MRI successfully identified the glioblastomatous component within a surrounding region of solid tumor tissue otherwise interpreted as an anaplastic astrocytoma. Two patients with enhancing old peritumoral hemorrhage were successfully biopsied when PET demonstrated focal nodules of metastatic carcinoma that were obscured from CT and MRI. One patient was suspected of having an intracranial abscess because of intense hypometabolism within a ring enhancing lesion that suggested a metastasis on CT and MRI, which proved to be a correct predictor of histology.

PET-FDG images can be successfully incorporated into routine image-directed stereotactic surgery. Stereotactic biopsy sampling of intracranial masses is more likely to produce diagnostically valid results when directed by correlative imaging that includes the functional information of PET-FDG data.

References

1 Sokoloff L, Reivich M, Kennedy C, Des Rosiers M, Patlak C, Pettigrew K, Sakarada O, Shinohara M: The (14-C) deoxyglucose method for measurement of local cerebral glucose utilization: The theory, procedure, and normal values in conscious and anesthetized albino rat. J Neurochem 1977;28:897–916.

2 Phelps M, Huang S, Hoffman E, Selin C, Sokoloff L, Kuhl D: Tomographic measurement of local cerebral glucose metabolic rate in humans with (F-18) 2-fluoro-2-deoxy-*D*-glucose: Validation of method. Ann Neurol 1979;6:371–388.

3 Kelly P, Earnest F, Kall B, Goerss S, Scheithauer B: Surgical options for patients with deep-seated brain tumors: Computer-assisted stereotactic biopsy. Mayo Clin Proc 1985;60:223–229.

Robert J. Maciunas, MD, Department of Neurosurgery, T 4224 MCN,
Vanderbilt University Medical Center, Nashville, TN 37232 (USA).

Proceedings of the Meeting of the American Society for Stereotactic and Functional Neurosurgery, Pittsburgh, Pa., June 16–19, 1991
Stereotact Funct Neurosurg 1992;58:141–143

Three-Dimensional Whole-Brain Mapping

T.L. Hardy, L.R.D. Brynildson, J.G. Gray, D. Spurlock
University of New Mexico School of Medicine, Albuquerque, N.Mex., USA

Key Words. Computer · Stereotactic surgery · Brain mapping · Three-dimensional brain imaging

Abstract. The implementation and use of a computerized whole-brain mapping system which can be used in conjunction with MRI, CT, angiographic and other brain imaging techniques is described. Three mapping systems based upon common reference structures about the third and fourth ventricular core of the brain are used in conjunction with internationally recognized nomenclature to create a normalized whole-brain mapping system according to the Talairach/Tournoux proportional grid technique.

The use of brain mapping techniques has been important in the development of stereotaxy. Historically, static atlas maps consisting of tracings of anatomic microscopic sections of the brain cut in orthogonal planes have been used as an index of stereotactic anatomic topography [1–3]. Additionally, electrophysiological maps, determined from preoperative recordings and stimulation of the brain, have also been utilized by various authors [1–7]. Talairach and Tournoux [7] pioneered the method of creating a normalized proportional grid of the whole brain, so that the structures most likely to be found in a given voxel of the brain could be determined. This method has been noted by others to be reasonably reliable in discerning brain anatomic topography [8]. Each of these works have been distinct entities with little cross-correlation between the information they contain, other than their use of common brain reference structures for either creating anatomic static maps or proportional grids. With modern computer imaging and

1011–6125/92/0584–0141 $ 2.75/0

graphics techniques, it is possible to create large data bases containing the information in the various mapping systems noted above for composite display, cross-referencing and also mapping of information known or acquired by other mapping techniques.

Our original brain mapping techniques [4–6] have been expanded so that MR and CT images can be displayed in a three-dimensionally simulated stereotactic frame environment. Various combinations of MR images as well as CT images (or combinations of both and angiography) can be selectively displayed and viewed in three-dimensional stereotactic space. The Talairach/Tournoux [7] whole-brain proportional voxel technique of statistically determining the most likely anatomic structures in a voxel of brain of a given patient has been developed in conjunction with this technique to map any given area of the brain (fig. 1). Data from the Talairach/Tournoux anatomic library, the architectonics of Van Buren and Borke, Schaltenbrand and Bailey, Schaltenbrand and Wahren [1–3], and Brodmann [1–3, 7, 8] have been used to develop a detailed anatomic atlas library. The data in this mapping and imaging environment can be interrogated to create computerized anatomic displays (fig. 1, 2) showing any given functional anatomic region in two-dimensional displays or three-dimensional relief.

The interrogation and cross-referencing of data from various brain mapping systems is possible in this normalized whole-brain mapping technique (fig. 1, 2). It is also useful for determining anatomic sites of probe trajectories for morphological and functional procedures, radiation dosimetry to anatomic sites, identification of anatomic sites of various responses obtained with electromagnetic encephalography and standard EEG, cross-correlation of metabolic anatomico-topographical imaging, and the interrogation and cross-referencing of imaging data by various digital imaging techniques.

References

1 Van Buren JM, Borke RC: Variations and Connections of the Human Thalamus. New York, Springer, 1972, vol 1 and 2.

2 Schaltenbrand G, Bailey P: Introduction to Stereotaxis with an Atlas of the Human Brain. New York, Thieme, 1959.

3 Schaltenbrand G, Wahren W: Atlas for Stereotaxy of the Human Brain, ed 2. Stuttgart, Thieme, 1977.

4 Hardy TL: Stereotactic CT atlases; in Lunsford LD (ed): Modern Stereotactic Surgery. Boston, Nijhoff, 1988, chapt 34.

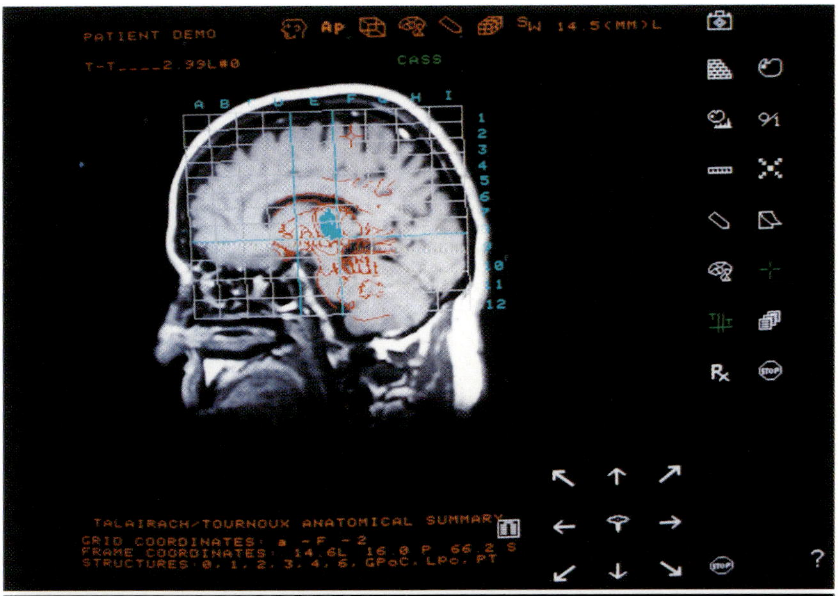
PATIENT DEMO
AP
SW 14.5(MM)L
T-T____2.99L#0
CASS
TALAIRACH/TOURNOUX ANATOMICAL SUMMARY
GRID COORDINATES: a - F - 2
FRAME COORDINATES: 14.6L 16.0 P 66.2 S
STRUCTURES: 0, 1, 2, 3, 4, 6, GPoC, LPo, PT
Rx
STOP
?

1

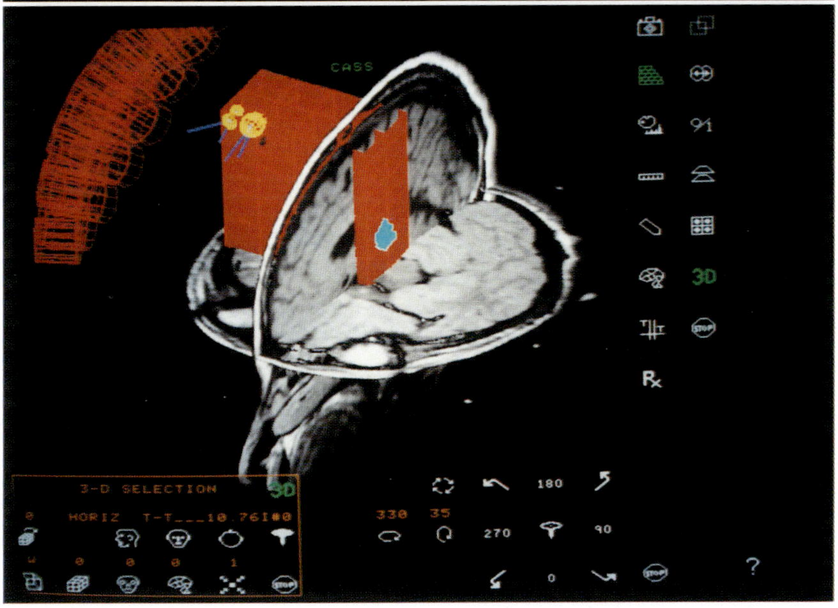
CASS
3D
Rx
STOP
3-D SELECTION
HORIZ T-T___10.76I#0
180
330 35
270
90
0
?

2

Fig. 1. Sagittal MR image with composite overlay of scaled Schaltenbrand and Wahren [3] diencephalic and brainstem map which has nonevoked rhythmic cellular responses [4, 5] to microelectrode recordings plotted in the region of ventralis intermedius. The Talairach/Tournoux [7] proportional grid is also overlayed and a cursor is positioned in voxel of sensory/motor strip area. Computer printout of Talairach/Tournoux grid coordinates, stereotactic frame coordinates and anatomic brain structures, and Brodmann's areas for voxel of cursor's position are noted below.

Fig. 2. Three-dimensional display of sagittal and horizontal MR images in stereotactic frame space showing position of sensory/motor strip (red) and nonevoked rhythmic responses (blue area) in graphic relief. Position of dipole moment for finger impulses on EMEG recording is seen as sphere (yellow) over motor strip area. Squid EMEG array is simulated in upper left corner.

5 Hardy TL: A method for MRI and CT mapping of diencephalic somatotopography. Stereotact Funct Neurosurg 1989;52:242–249.
6 Hardy TL, Brynildson LRD: Computer rendering of stereotactic atlas data and whole brain mapping with computed tomography and magnetic resonance imaging; in Kelly PJ (ed): Computers in Stereotactic Neurosurgery. New York, Blackwell, 1990.
7 Talairach J, Tournoux P: Co-Planar Stereotaxic Atlas of Human Brain: 3-Dimensional Proportional System. New York, Thieme, 1988.
8 Steinmetz H, Furst G, Freund JH: Cerebral cortical localization: Application and validation of the proportional grid system in MR imaging. J Comput Assist Tomogr 1989;13:10–19.

T.L. Hardy, MD, Neurosurgery Department, Lovelace Medical Center,
5400 Gibson Blvd. SE, Albuquerque, NM 87108 (USA)

Proceedings of the Meeting of the American Society for Stereotactic and Functional Neurosurgery, Pittsburgh, Pa., June 16–19, 1991
Stereotact Funct Neurosurg 1992;58:144–152

A Stereotactic Digitizing Arm

S.J. Goerss, P.J. Kelly, B.A. Kall, S.O. Stiving
Department of Neurosurgery, Mayo Clinic, Rochester, Minn., USA

Our group has been working on the development of a stereotactic system to provide a versatile unit to perform a variety of procedures. The positioner, primarily designed to resect deep-seated tumors and to perform stereotactic biopsies, has evolved over a period of years with the goal to extend its use in other types of stereotactic procedures. A natural by-product of the software and instrumentation is its application in the resection of superficially located tumors. The use of stereotaxy for these procedures was overlooked due to the relative ease of the procedures. However, stereotaxy can be an important asset for these procedures as well. Using the treatment-planning software, the location, size and orientation of the lesion is determined. A display of the tumor volume is made with a representation of trephine overlayed. From this, the surgeon can predetermine the smallest-size trephine required to expose the tumor and center it directly over the lesion. Intraoperatively, the trephine is used to relate the boundary of the tumor in the surgical field. The dimension that is lost is the depth of the surgical field which, in most cases, is the most critical. To better utilize the data base and maintain quantitative control of the procedure, a digitizing arm has been incorporated into the stereotactic system. Software has been developed which relates the location of the distal end of the arm to the patient's data base. Using the device, the surgeon may point to an area of the surgical field and determine the relationship between the pointer and the stereotactic CT, MRI, DSA or reconstructed volumetric tumor cross-sections. This approach maintains the surgeon's orientation as the procedure progresses.

Stereotactic Neurosurgical Operating Arm System

B.L. Guthrie, R. Kaplan, D. Florek
Department of Neurosurgery, George Washington University,
Washington, D.C., USA

In an effort to broaden the range of stereotaxy to include standard neurosurgical cases, we have developed the Stereotactic Operating Arm System, a frameless stereotactic system based on a multijointed passively moved operating arm coupled to a computer. Calibration of the system is accomplished using 3 non-colinear scalp markers (skin staples) placed anywhere on the head prior to a preoperative CT scan. In the operating room, the Operating Arm is attached to the operating table and calibrated to

1011–6125/92/0584–0144 $ 2.75/0

the CT scan using the 3 scalp points after the patient is placed in the desired operative position. Presurgical planning involves the surgeon moving the Arm around the head while the computer simultaneously displays localization information in a variety of formats. The location of the tip of the arm can be shown on axial CT slices, any planar reconstruction of the head (cut-away-views) and on a three-dimensional reconstruction of the head. Several trajectory displays, including 'multiple slice', planar reconstruction and an 'arms-eye-view', show the surgeon what lies ahead of the Arm tip. Once the operation is underway, these views help keep the surgeon oriented and apprised of his operative location to an accuracy of 2.5 mm. Intraoperatively, the arm may be used as a 'three-dimensional' mouse to control program flow via menus such that no keyboard input is required. The Operative Arm System has been used for approximately 50 cases, including subdural hematomas, meningiomas, astrocytomas and placement of ventricular catheters, expanding the range of computer-assisted localization to standard neurosurgical procedures. Throughout this project, we have repeatedly found that it is exceedingly difficult to depict three-dimensional information on two-dimensional medium for surgical purposes. We continue to strive to optimize the use of digital imaging data in an interactive fashion for cranial procedures.

An Arc-Radius, Rectilinear Stereotactic System with Particular Application in Functional Neurosurgery

M.P. Carol, J.A. Brown
Route 1, Melford, N.Y., USA

The 'gNomos' is an arc-radius, variable linear offset, skull-mounted stereotactic system. By virtue of its design, it is compact, simple to understand and use, and supports certain applications not possible with other systems. One of these applications is in the field of functional procedures. The targets for many of these procedures are referenced to the anterior-posterior commissure (AC-PC) line, as are the standard physiological and anatomic atlases. With most current stereotactic systems, the approximate target point can be generated from either CT or MRI. However, physiologic verification based on anatomic parameters is usually needed prior to lesioning. This requires offsetting the target in the x, y and/or z directions until the precise lesion location is identified. In current systems, this offsetting occurs in a plane parallel to the frame which secures the system to the patient's skull, a plane perpendicular to the imaging table. Consequently, although the patient can be imaged parallel to the AC-PC line by appropriate angulation of the gantry, the offsetting which occurs is not in this plane. It is therefore not in the plane of the anatomic and physiological atlases, introducing guess work into determining the final site of lesioning. gNomos allows the plane in which the offsets occur to be varied (variable linear offset capability). The system, once mounted on the patient's skull, can be angulated, allowing it to be brought parallel to the plane of the AC-PC line. Once the approximate target point has been identified, offsets can be referenced both physiologically and anatomically to standard atlases to find the exact point where the lesion is to be made. This eliminates much of the guess work involved, reducing the number of passes of the simulating electrode which might otherwise be required.

Stereotactic Craniotomy Using the Brown-Roberts-Wells System

R.J. Maciunas
Department of Neurological Surgery, Vanderbilt University Medical Center, Nashville, Tenn., USA

Precise localization of subcortical targets contributes to the technical challenge of craniotomies. To address this challenge using commonly available equipment, the CT-compatible Brown-Roberts-Wells (BRW) stereotactic apparatus was evaluated as a guidance technique. Over a 3-year period, 100 consecutive stereotactic craniotomies were performed successfully using standard BRW hardware and software. This included 81 craniotomies in 68 patients for resection of subcortical mass lesions, and 19 cases of adrenal medullary transplantation for movement disorders. The average age of 59 male and 28 female patients was 48.5 years. Targets were consistently and precisely localized by the stereotactic frame. Mass lesions were frontal (3%), frontoparietal (24%), parietal (21%), occipitoparietotemporal (15%), temporal (8%), occipital (15%), basal ganglia/internal capsule (13%), thalamic (3%) and cerebellar (3%). All 19 adrenal transplantations targeted the right dorsomedial periventricular caudate. Gross total resection of all solid tumor tissue was consistently confirmed by postoperative contrasted CT. Average resected tumor volume was 55,903 mm^3. Pathology included metastases (52%), glial tumors (29%), nonglial tumors (8%) and nonneoplastic lesions (11%). Histology differed in 24.6% from presumptive neurodiagnostic imaging diagnoses. Postoperatively, 61% of patients with masses improved neurologically, 35.5% were unchanged and 3.5% worsened. Preoperative Karnofsky scores averaged 71; postoperatively, 63% were improved, 35% were unchanged and 2% worsened. Four transplantation patients improved; none worsened. There were no postoperative deaths. Overall surgical morbidity for mass lesion resection was 3.7%. This included worsened right hemiparesis after resection of a left rolandic glioblastoma, worsened left-hand monoparesis after resection of an internal capsule metastasis, and superior quadrantanopsia after an occipital oligodendroglioma resection. One asymptomatic sterile abscess occurred within the corticotomy after adrenal transplantation. Median postoperative survival for glioblastoma was 58.7 weeks and for metastases, 39.2 weeks. There were no complications referable to stereotactic localization. Hospitalization averaged 6 days. CT-directed stereotactic craniotomy using the BRW system is a safe, efficacious and readily available technique. It successfully confers the precision of stereotactic methodology onto open microneurosurgical procedures.

Stereotactic Approach to the Tumors in and around the Cavernous Sinus

A. Patil, P. Kumar, L. Leibrock
Division of Neurosurgery, University of Nebraska
Medical Center, Omaha, N. Dak, USA

Open surgical approaches to the cavernous sinus are considered difficult and dangerous because of the close proximity of vital neural and vascular structures. Modern imaging modalities like CT and MR scans provide the surgeon with images of structures in this area and make it possible to combine these imaging modalities with stereotaxis in order to provide safe trajectory in reaching this area. Stereotactic approach was used for placement of high-intensity [^{125}I]-seeds in 10 patients because open surgery was refused (1), or the patient's health did not permit open surgery (1), or total surgical resection was unsuccessful (2), or the tumor was recurrent (6). The tumors were either in the anterior third (1), or the middle third (2) or the posterior third (3), or involving more than one segment of the cavernous sinus (4). The pathology of the tumors were meningioma (7), chondrosarcoma (1) and metastases (2). Coronal, sagittal and axial MR and axial CT images were used to plan trajectories that would avoid critical neural and vascular structures. The procedures were performed under local anesthesia with intraoperative CT scan monitoring. One to 3 high-intensity ^{125}-I-seeds were placed in the tumor using a 16-gauge needle. The hospital stay was 24 h. No acute complications resulted. The median for follow-up is 12 months, the longest being 35 months. Tumor regression was seen in all 8 patients who had longer than 3 months follow-up, with 80–100% regression in 7 of them. One-patient had progression of fifth cranial nerve involvement 8 months after the procedure and another had transient involvement of the third cranial nerve 3 months after the procedure. Both these patients have metastatic lesions. In summary, the cavernous sinus can be approached safely using stereotactic technique for the purpose of brachytherapy and could prove useful in the treatment of unresectable lesions in the cavernous sinus.

Comparison between MRI- and CT-Scan-Guided Stereotactic Biopsy

A. De Salles, D. Mock, K. Black, D. Becker
Division of Neurosurgery, UCLA Medical Center, Los Angeles, Calif., USA

MRI-guided stereotactic biopsy was performed in 12 patients with an intracranial mass lesions. There were 4 brainstem and 8 supratentorial lesions. A Fonar 0.3-tesla scanner, GE-9800 CT scanner, and a Brown-Roberts-Wells stereotactic system were used. The needle trajectory was planned having the skull entry point anteroposterior and vertical coordinates derived from a sagittal cut and the lateral coordinate derived from a coronal cut. The progression of the needle throughout the tumor was also planned in advance. The Euclidean distances between the target point as determined on axial, coronal and sagittal MRI scans and on an axial CT scan cut were compared. The biopsy was diagnostic in 11 of the 12 patients. There were 5 glioblastoma multiforme, 3 astrocytomas grade III, 2 astrocytomas grade II, 1 metastatic melanoma and 1 was a negative biopsy. This last patient had an enlarged left brachium conjunctivum and mesencephalon without contrast enhancement either on the MRI or on the CT scan. He was also the only patient who presented a new neurological symptom possibly related to the biopsy. He developed a thalamic pain syndrome 3 weeks after the procedure. The mean Euclidean distance between targets determined on the different planes was 12.1 mm, the range was from 1.3 to 32.6 mm. No attempt was made to repeat the target in each cartesian plane. The optimal diagnostic target in each plane was chosen. Therefore, the distances between target points do not represent the technique accuracy, instead it represents different perspectives of the same mass lesion. When comparing target distances plane by plane, the axial versus sagittal distance was 11.7 ± 6.9 mm, the sagittal versus coronal was 12.8 ± 5.6 mm, the axial versus coronal was 10.8 ± 8.2 mm, the axial MRI versus axial CT scan was 11.2 ± 10.0 mm, the sagittal MRI versus axial CT scan was 14.8 ± 9.5 mm, and the coronal MRI versus axial CT scan was 12.3 ± 6.1 mm. MRI-guided stereotactic biopsy offers direct visualization of the target in three dimensions coupled with a detailed anatomy of the needle trajectory. Targets derived from axial, sagittal and coronal cuts not always are close in distance from each other. By interchanging coordinates derived from the three cartesian planes, one can optimize targeting and increase the safety of the procedure.

Stereotactic Endoscopic Resection of Intraaxial and Intraventricular Brain Tumors Using High-Power Lasers

T. Otsuki, T. Yoshimoto, H. Jokura, S. Saso
Division of Neurosurgery, Institute of Brain Diseases,
Tohoku University School of Medicine, Sendai, Japan

A new stereotactic endoscopic approach is presented using both high-power lasers and fine microsurgical techniques to resect deep-seated solid lesions through a guiding tube of 8 mm. Since the operating field is kept dry and exposed to the air, this endoscopic system can be regarded as an open system. The guiding tube is adapted to the standard Leksell stereotactic apparatus and inserted stereotactically to the target through a burr hole. At the target point, the inner stylet is removed and either a rigid or flexible endoscope is inserted for visualization. Various flexible microsurgical instruments, such as suction tubes, tumor forceps, dissectors or scissors, can be inserted through the side window of the guiding tube and manipulated. Nd:Yag laser is transmitted through a quartz fiber inserted into a flexible metal tube. Massive gas produced by laser irradiation is aspirated to maintain the clear vision. A surgeon can aspirate, dissect and remove the lesions using these instruments and also apply cotton pledgets and other hemostatic materials to control bleeding with irrigation and suction. Twenty-two intraaxial lesions were operated on by this approach, in which 10 small (3–26 mm) tumors were totally removed without significant complications. Contact Yag laser tips were particularly effective for tissue vaporization whereas noncontact tips were useful for coagulation and hemostasis. Stereotactic open-system endoscopy only requires a small burr hole at the skull to approach the operating field, thus causing minimum damage to the normal brain. Intraoperative displacement of the targeted lesions is also minimized in this surgery, so that accurate resection of pathological lesions according to the presurgical planning based on CT/MR images can be achieved.

CT-Guided Stereotactic Biopsy Using the Pelorus System A Critical Appraisal

H.H. Engelhard, G.B. Nazar
University of Louisville, Kent., USA

The Pelorus stereotactic system has been promoted as being a simple and inexpensive system for use in performing CT-guided stereotactic brain biopsy. Although the system has been available for 6 years, very little infomation about its use and diagnostic accuracy has been reported in the literature. Objections to using the system have centered on its limited flexibility and its possible lack of precision in localizing lesions within the brain. This study presents the results obtained with 20 consecutive patients who underwent CT-guided stereotactic biopsy using the Pelorus apparatus. The patients ranged from 7 months to 79 years of age. Ten patients were male and 10 female. Eleven patients were 16 years of age or younger. Sixteen biopsies were performed under general anesthesia, while 4 were performed under local anesthesia. Anatomically, the system was primarily used to localize deep-seated lesions within the cerebral hemispheres. Pathological diagnosis was obtained in 17 out of 20 patients. In 2 out of the 17 cases diagnosed by biopsy, infection was the etiology. The remaining patients were found to have various types of tumors. In the 3 cases not diagnosed by biopsy, tumor was subsequently found to be present. In 1 case, tumor seeding was later noted to occur along the biopsy track. The authors conclude that the ability of the Pelorus system to obtain diagnostic tissue compares favorably with other stereotactic systems. The system was found to be particularly useful in the pediatric age group, although its use in very young patients requires special adaptations. The main limitation of the system, when used for biopsy, is in its ability to reach multiple targets. In certain settings, the Pelorus system may be useful, as a lower-cost alternative to conventional stereotactic frames, for obtaining CT-guided brain biopsy.

A Neurosurgical Image-Guided Localizing Unit for Open Stereotaxis

L. Zamorano, M. Dujovny, C.M. Chavantes
Department of Neurosurgery, University Health Center, Detroit, Mich., USA

A unit was developed to provide the neurosurgeon with a CT-, MRI-, DA-compatible head holder and image localization as well as freedom of choice for surgical approach and patient's intraoperative positioning (ZD Multipurpose Neurosurgical Localizing Unit, Fischer, Freiburg, FRG). The unit consists of a CT-, MRI- and DA-compatible carbon fiber ring-shaped head holder with special features of free selection for fixations's point, avoiding interference with the flap site or craniotomy. A CT, MRI and DA adaptation allows easy measurement of coordinates on any of these image modalities. The base ring is mounted intraoperatively on a Mayfield or Sugita adapter allowing any positioning of the patient: supine, lateral, prone, 3/4 prone, sitting, etc. Surgical draping gives a completely sterile field. An arc-quadrant-localizing aiming device is mounted on any alternative 4 positions according to the neurosurgeon' preference; x, y and z coordinates are adjusted directly; 2 angles define the precalculated trajectory, and the instrument holder adjusts the depth. A PC-compatible software gives the settings for any possible mounting in order to achieve the same trajectory. Intraoperatively, the localizing system can be used in a 'fixed' permanent setting, or as a 'nonfixed' system just to provide intraoperative three-dimensional orientation. In the first case, which corresponds to a more conventional stereotactic approach, different arc-adapted instrumentation gives the unit further capabilities, especially 'bayonet'-type brain retractors and endoscopes. In the case of a nonfixed setting, the system provides the benefit of intraoperative accurate orientation and use of conventional neuromicrosurgical techniques without mechanical obstruction; in this case self-retaining retractor arms are fixed to the ring including flexible arms; brain spatules are used on the stereotactic microsurgical resection of deep lesions. Intraoperative imaging localization, such as DA, is also possible. Unit details, methodology and clinical experience in 203 consecutive cases of open stereotactic surgery will be presented.

Computer-Assisted Neurosugery: Simulation and Automation

L. Zamorano, M. Dujovny, A. Dong, M. Kadi
Department of Neurosurgery, University Health Center, Detroit, Mich., USA

The introduction of computers in neurosurgery has opened a new frontier allowing the neurosurgeon simulation, optimization and automation for resection of intracranial lesions. A system and methodology for computer-assisted neurosurgery (CAN) is presented. Tomographic (CT, MRI or projective DA) images are acquired with a fixed carbon fiber base ring (Z/D Localizing unit, Fisher, Freiburg, FRG). The image data are loaded into a workstation (SUN 4/370) for simulation and optimization of the surgical procedure performed using a specially designed software and hardware configuration: Neurosurgical Stereotactic Planning System (NSPS). The software of the NSPS system includes module for two- and three-dimensional image reconstruction stereotactic conditions; multiple approaches can be simulated and optimized and once the surgical approach has been elected on a special mode, 'surgeon's perspective', generate multiformated two-dimensional display of free tilt reformatted images perpendicular to the selected trajectory of the entire target volume at desired intervals. A file is created that contains the boundaries of resection at each level of the surgeon's perspective. This file can be transferred to the operating room in two specific ways: (1) through a special image board into video images that are displayed by a specially developed optical mechanism into the surgeon's eyepiece of the automated microscope, and (2) the same file is transferred as digital information through either network to a computer driving the automated microscope to control the movements of the microscope and laser joystick console. At the level of the operating room, the surgeon operates a friendly menu-driven software with the Microscope Remote Controller (MIRC) which consists of a PC-based, 3-access motor controller, indexer and driver; this controls a high accurate rate digital brushless motor which is fixed in the microscope. The software at this level allows the surgeon to use the travel control that moves the microscope along the surgical trajectory. At the same time, the appropriate boundary of the lesion is displayed at each level of the movement and projects into the microscope to guide the surgeon through the lesion's resection. Finally, an automated laser resection system is provided using as input the same digital file that controls the automated microscope. The PC is connected to the laser remote control through a specially designed circuit that emulates the joystick function, and the software coordinates the movement of the microscope, allowing the preplanned trajectory (z direction) with the movement of the microscan laser beam (x, y direction). In summary, a system for CAN has been developed using a central multitasking Unix-based computer system which allows simulation, optimization and automated movement of the computer-control-based microscope and laser joystick console.

Stereotactic Endoscopy

L. Zamorano, C. Chavantes, M. Dujovny, J.I. Ausman
Department of Neurosurgery, University Health Center,
Detroit, Mich., USA

Endoscopic laser stereotaxis (ELS) involves integration of rigid-flexible endoscopy and Nd:YAG laser to three-/two-dimensional multiplaner image-guided stereotactic procedures. The major advantages of ELS include: direct intraoperative visualization, hemostasis, evacuation or resection assessment, and wide exploration of intracranial cavities or ventricles. The technique allows safe aspiration, biopsy and resection or internal decompression of deep cystic and intraventricular lesions. With adequate methodology, the stereotactic technique achieves 1 mm accuracy on both the x and y axis and 1.5 mm in the z axis. Nevertheless, major criticisms and limitations of 'nonresective' image-guided stereotaxis have been the lack of direct visualization and intraoperative monitoring of the procedures, morbidity and mortality due to hemorrhages associated with intraoperative blindness, and changes in intracranial coordinates after aspiration of cystic cavities or intraventricular lesions. To overcome some of these limitations in addition to increasing the scope of clinical usefulness of image guidance to a wider range of intracranial pathology, we have adapted flexible and rigid endoscopy and Nd:YAG laser to stereotaxis. Main indications have included cystic intraaxial (tumors, hematomas, benign cysts, abscess, etc.) and intraventricular lesions. The basic ELS instrumentation includes: endoscopic instrumentation (rigid-flexible), stereotactic frames (Riechert-Mundinger, Zamorano-Dujovny) and a cannula adapter for stereotactic arc. Rigid neuroendoscopy is performed by a 6-mm cannula and a zero degree rigid optics (Stroz, Culver City, Calif., USA). Endoscopic rigid instrumentation includes different biopsy forceps (punch cup, alligator, etc.), hook scissors and bipolar coagulating electrodes. Fiberoptic neuroendoscopy is performed with a flexible Olympus fiber endoscope (ENT-1T10; Olympus, Strongsville, Ohio, USA) and flexible instrumentation similar to the rigid endoscope. A videocamera and a beamsplitter allows simultaneous display on the optics and television monitor. A 1.8-mm Nd:YAG laser disposable fiber (SLT, Malvern, Pa., USA) is introduced through the 2-mm channels of both rigid and flexible endoscopes. The Nd:YAG laser (Cooper 1800, MBB) can be used in conventional noncontact technique or with contact laser probes. Clinical experience in 80 consecutive cases will be presented. Also a new prototype of stereotactic neuroendoscope will be presented.

Epilepsy

Proceedings of the Meeting of the American Society for Stereotactic and Functional Neurosurgery, Pittsburgh, Pa., June 16–19, 1991
Stereotact Funct Neurosurg 1992;58:153–161

Intraoperative Brain Mapping Techniques in Neuro-Oncology

Mitchel S. Berger, George A. Ojemann

Department of Neurological Surgery, University of Washington School of Medicine, Northwest Neuro-Oncology Research and Therapy Section, Seattle, Wash., USA

Key Words. Brain mapping · Gliomas · Speech areas · Motor pathways · Seizures

Abstract. Intraoperative brain mapping techniques are utilized in neuro-oncology to maximize the extent of tumor resection and seizure control, and minimize the operative morbidity. Direct stimulation mapping of the cortex and subcortical descending motor pathways will localize the rolandic cortex, dominant language speech zones and motor tracts in the internal capsule, cerebral peduncle and corticospinal tract/anterior horn cells. Electrocorticography identifies epileptogenic areas that histologically are distinctly devoid of neoplastic infiltration. Seizure control is maximal when seizure foci are resected in addition to the tumor nidus.

Recently, the rationale for radical resection of intrinsic brain and spinal cord tumors, as a prelude to more aggressive adjuvant therapy, has been reassessed. Evidence supports the approach that a more extensive malignant tumor removal favorably influences the time to tumor progression and survival, while often improving the functional status of the patient [1–3]. This is, in part, explained by the local recurrence patterns of these tumors following radical resection. In Wallner et al.'s recent series [4], the majority of tumors (81%) recurred locally within 2.0 cm of the margins of the resection cavity. Although somewhat more controversial of an issue with low-grade gliomas, emphasis on radical resection, especially when combined with focal postoperative radiotherapy, is gaining support. This is based on data from several retrospective studies analyzing the time to tumor progression and survival as a function of extent of tumor resection [5, 6]. Although not analyzed in the previous literature, it would be interesting to speculate whether radical resection for low-grade gliomas affects the recurrence pattern in terms of the histological phenotype, e.g. less likely to have a malignant recurrence with a more aggressive resection. This is currently under retrospective evaluation at our institution.

Intractable epilepsy associated with low-grade gliomas in children and young adults constitutes an additional indication for an operative procedure designed to map and resect seizure foci. Because these epileptogenic zones are usually separated from the tumor nidus [7], the combined tumor plus functional resection cavity may, necessarily, become quite extensive. We agree with other investigators that removing the tumor without resecting the seizure foci may yield less than optimal results when control of tumor-associated epilepsy is an important factor [8, 9].

Therefore, when considering the relevant issues of modern-day glioma surgery, it becomes imperative to utilize currently available methodology to safely achieve the goals of maximal tumor resection and seizure control. Intraoperative stimulation mapping and electrocorticography have been used for many years for epilepsy surgery to identify language, motor and sensory regions, in addition to defining seizure foci [10–12]. At the University of Washington, in conjunction with our Regional Epilepsy Center and Functional Brain Mapping Program, we have adapted these techniques to enhance the surgery of intrinsic brain and spinal cord tumors.

Materials and Methods

Rationale

Tumors adjacent to or involving regions associated with language, motor or sensory function are suitable for intraoperative mapping. This includes the posterior frontal and anterior parietal region abutting the rolandic cortex, dominant-hemisphere language zones in the temporal, frontal and parietal areas, and any region with close proximity to the descending motor tracts, e.g. insula, corona radiata and internal capsule. Mesial temporal tumors with extension into the temporal stem will often obscure the normal anatomy of the incisura, therefore stimulation to identify the cerebral peduncle is particularly useful (fig. 1). Enough experience has been gained during intramedullary tumor removal to recommend this technique to identify either the corticospinal tract or anterior horn cells. The stimulation current is markedly different, e.g. 0.5–2 mA, from that used to map cortical or subcortical pathways (2–16 mA).

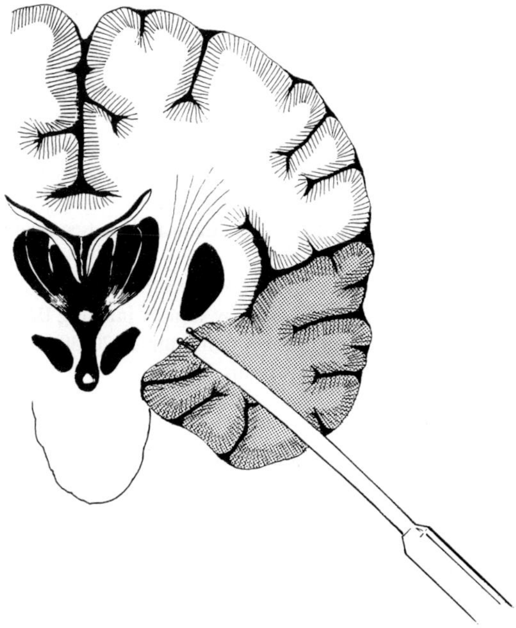

Fig. 1. Bipolar stimulator positioned at the mesial temporal lobe to identify the descending motor tracts of the cerebral peduncle.

When the tumor is associated with difficult to medically control seizure activity, intraoperative electrocorticography (ECoG) is a useful adjunct. At times, due to the age of the patient or their cooperative status, a subdural electrode array may be inserted 1 week prior to the definitive tumor removal to map seizure foci, in addition to functional cortical regions. Strip electrodes should be placed under the temporal lobe in several locations, e.g., anterior, middle and posterior, to identify inferior and mesial seizure foci. Because the epileptogenic zones are often adjacent to the lesion and devoid of neoplastic infiltration, postresection ECoG is necessary to verify that no significant seizure foci remain.

Caveats

Children less than 5 years of age often have electrically inexcitable cortex in terms of eliciting motor responses from direct stimulation under general anesthesia. This is often overcome by stimulating the surface, while awake on the hospital ward, using the subdural electrode array. However, if this is not possible, intraoperative evoked potentials may be used to identify the central sulcus via a phase reversal potential. Unfortunately, subcortical motor pathways cannot be identified using this latter technology.

Wada testing [13] should be used in any circumstance where cerebral dominance for speech is unclear, e.g. left-handedness. If speech function, reading and comprehension are impaired due to the location of the tumor, awake intraoperative testing will often not yield useful data and, thus, should not be performed. The anesthetic condition of the patient should be evaluated prior to motor mapping. Complete reversal of the paralytic agent is mandatory and may often be evaluated by applying the bipolar electrode to depolarize the exposed temporalis or occipital muscles, prior to cortical stimulation.

If the patient's seizures are well controlled on anticonvulsants, it is unlikely that significant interictal activity will be identified during surgery. Ideally, the patient should be poorly controlled on maximal medical therapy at the time of surgery. Chemical activation of epileptiform discharges may be evoked by rapidly infusing Brevital (1 mg/kg) intravenously. ECoG should be performed for a minimum of 20–30 min to ensure an adequate time period to evaluate epileptiform discharges.

Mapping Techniques

For awake craniotomies the scalp is widely anesthetized using a 0.5% lidocaine and 0.25% marcaine mixture. A large scalp and bone flap is necessary to allow for exposure of the tumor, functional zones and adjacent epileptogenic foci.

Following ultrasound localization of the tumor, the motor cortex is identified by stimulating the surface with a bipolar electrode (tips spaced 5 mm apart) in the region of the rolandic area [14]. A constant-current generator is used to produce a train of biphasic square wave pulses. The pulse frequency is 60 Hz with a single phase duration of 1 ms. The bipolar tips remain in place for 1–3 s and the optimal current will vary depending upon the anesthetic condition of the patient, e.g. 2–16 mA. The bipolar electrode should be applied parallel to the sulcus adjacent to the gyrus to be stimulated. Under general anesthesia the face motor area may be more difficult to elicit stimulation responses from and often requires a higher-range current. Any time a movement is witnessed, the surface that is stimulated should be marked with a numbered ticket. During the tumor resection the same current may be applied to the subcortical region to localize descending motor tracts. When stimulating in this area, the entire opposite extremity, including the face, should be viewed to identify any or all responses. Based on correlation of postoperative scans with stimulation-induced motor responses, and cortical sites of activation with quantification of distances at adjacent sites without responses, very little current spread, e.g. less than 2 mm, occurs even at higher milliampere levels. Brief motor seizures may occur and usually dissipate within 30 s.

ECoG is performed using a standard array of carbon-tipped electrodes attached to a horseshoe clamp and placed on the brain surface adjacent to the mass. Strip electrodes under the temporal or frontal lobe are also inserted. Each electrode is numbered and charted on a corresponding schematic brain map. Following recording of epileptiform discharges, the electrodes are left in place and a small current (2–8 mA) is applied to a cortical zone directly in contact with the electrode. This will often evoke brief after-discharge potentials, thus yielding the desired current, e.g. the highest current that did not evoke more than a few or no after-discharge potentials, for language mapping.

The patient is presented with slides that require naming objects, e.g. 'This is a *cat* (picture of a cat)'. Repetitive (3 or more) errors in naming or anomia are documented during the stimulation process at each numbered cortical site. Complete speech arrest will localize Broca's area which is contiguous (anterior) to the face motor cortex.

Postresection ECoG is performed following tumor removal in all cases with breakthrough seizures preoperatively. It is especially important in the temporal lobe after the lesion is debulked and the exposed surface of the hippocampus is in view. Occasional epileptogenic foci different in configuration from the original activity or distant discharges (beyond 4–6 cm from the resection cavity) are not aggressively pursued.

Results

Cortical and Subcortical Motor Pathways

Following tumor resection the previously identified sites for motor function are restimulated to ensure that the pathways are still intact. When this is verified, the patient will not experience any permanent loss of motor function. However, if the resection cavity is very close to the motor tracts, temporary weakness is not unusual, and may last for several weeks postoperatively. Resection of tumors involving the supplementary motor area of either hemisphere produce a characteristic syndrome postoperatively [15]. This region is located at the posterior mesial border of the frontal lobe and is separated from the motor cortex by the premotor sulcus. A complete hemiplegia exists postoperatively, along with mutism if the dominant hemisphere is operated upon, and this resolves in a stepwise fashion beginning 1 or 2 weeks postoperatively. Complete return of function usually occurs within 4–16 weeks following surgery. This syndrome is important to recognize so the family and the patient may be counseled appropriately prior to surgery.

Language

In a previous publication from our group, we described the cortical localization of language in the dominant hemisphere of 117 patients [16]. These data revealed a large variability in speech localization within the Wernicke-Broca region. However, language sites were found outside of this anatomically traditional speech center. Naming errors have been documented to occur within 4 cm from the midline in the posterior frontal area and within the anterior portion of the temporal lobe. In another series of our patients retrospectively examined with dominant temporal lobe tumors, we found a 22% incidence of significant naming errors within 3 cm of the temporal lobe tip (fig. 2). In ad-

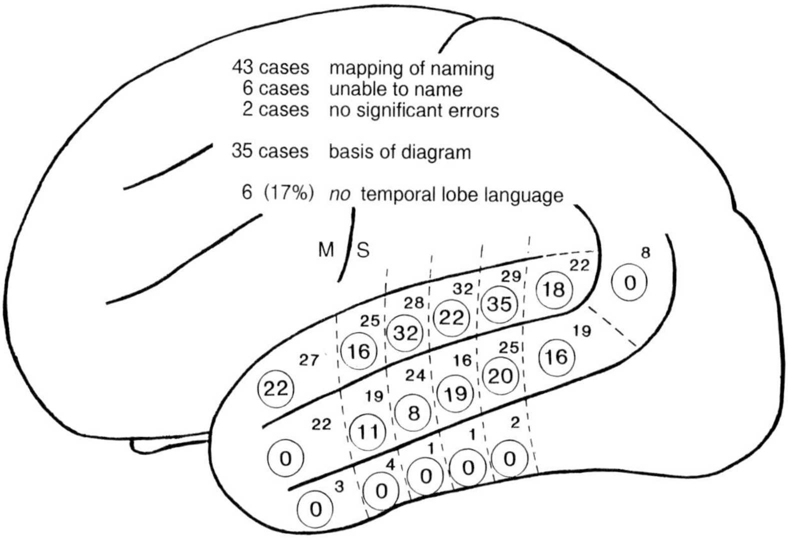

Fig. 2. Composite language map of patients with dominant temporal lobe tumors. The numbers inside the circles represent the percentage of language sites tested with repetitive naming errors. The numbers outside the circles indicate the number of sites tested. Seventeen percent of all these patients had no temporal lobe language sites. Speech representation was identified within 3 cm of the anterior temporal lobe tip in a significant number of cases.

dition, 17% of the 35 cases analyzed demonstrated no temporal lobe language sites.

When the resection cavity abuts the mapped-out speech areas, approximately 30–50% of the patients will have temporary language deficits according to the area resected, e.g. comprehension versus motor speech, which dissipates over weeks to a few months following surgery. Similar to the motor pathways, if speech is intact at the end of the procedure we expect full return of function without a permanent deficit. The temporary language problems are usually worse 48 h postoperatively when swelling is maximal.

Seizure Control

We recently reviewed a series of 46 adult and pediatric patients with low-grade gliomas and intractable epilepsy. All patients had therapeutic anticonvulsant levels using two or more antiepileptic drugs.

Fifty-eight seizure foci were detected in these 46 patients and, in 18 individuals, 2 anatomically distinct epileptogenic regions were identified. The majority of these (85%) foci were submitted for histology and in 90% of the specimens evaluated no tumor infiltration was present. Further analysis of tissue specimens from 4 patients revealed a statistically significant decrease in both somatostatin (74%) and GABAergic (51%) immunoreactive neurons in the epileptogenic cortex compared with the nonepileptogenic cortex from the same patient [M. Haglund, pers. commun.]. Patients with multiple seizure foci were more likely to have had a longer duration of their seizure activity than if only a single focus was identified. Overall, seizure control was better in pediatric patients following resection of tumor and electrocorticographically verified seizure foci, e.g. 93% of children were seizure-free off antiepileptic drugs at a mean of 24 months postoperatively. Although 85% of adult patients were seizure-free following surgery (mean follow-up, 27 months), only 62% of these patients were able to discontinue their medication completely. The remaining adults, however, had significantly reduced seizure frequency and severity on reduced levels of anticonvulsant drugs.

Discussion

Based on our experience using brain mapping techniques in over 270 patients with intrinsic tumors of the brain and spinal cord, we have been able to achieve a greater resection of the tumor and the infiltrated brain adjacent to the tumor nidus, improved seizure control, and less permanent operative morbidity. We prefer the direct stimulation methods originally described by Fritsch and Hitzig [17] and popularized by Penfield and Roberts [18] to map cortical and subcortical functional zones. We have avoided the use of somatosensory-evoked potentials to identify the rolandic cortex unless the patient is a young child. Relying on this method alone prevents the surgeon from being able to map descending motor pathways during the actual tumor resection.

Language localization is the most difficult aspect of the procedure as one must become familiar with valid language testing methods and recognize subtle changes in speech output, reading, comprehension and naming. Language is exquisitely variable in all individuals [16, 18] and is often not present where it is expected to be located. Finally, one can expect a greater degree of seizure control in pediatric patients. However, in either children or adults, seizure control is greatest when the tumor is removed in addition to distinct epileptiform foci, which are typically devoid of neoplastic infiltration.

Acknowledgements

This work was supported by the American Cancer Society Career Development Award and Clinical Professorship of Oncology, and NS01253-01 (M.S.B.) and NS17111, 21724 and 20482 (G.A.O.).

References

1 Ammirati M, Vick N, Liao Y, et al: Effect of the extent of surgical resection on survival and quality of life in patients with supratentorial glioblastomas and anaplastic astrocytomas. Neurosurgery 1987;21:201–206.

2 Ciric I, Ammirati M, Vick N, et al: Supratentorial gliomas: Surgical considerations and immediate postoperative results. Neurosurgery 1987;21:21–26.

3 Kelly PJ: Stereotactic biopsy and resection of thalamic astrocytomas. Neurosurgery 1989;25:185–194.

4 Wallner KE, Galicich JH, Krol G, et al: Patterns of failure following treatment for glioblastoma multiforme and anaplastic astrocytoma. Int J Radiat Oncol Biol Phys 1989;16:1405–1409.

5 Shaw EG, Daumas-Duport C, Scheithauer BW, et al: Radiation therapy and the management of low grade supratentorial astrocytomas. J Neurosurg 1989;70:853–861.

6 Soffieti R, Chio A, Giordina MT, et al: Prognostic factors in well differentiated cerebral astrocytomas in the adult. Neurosurgery 1989;24:686–692.

7 Berger MS, Kincaid J, Ojemann GA, et al: Brain mapping techniques to maximize resection, safety, and seizure control in children with brain tumors. Neurosurgery 1989;25:786–792.

8 Drake J, Hoffman HJ, Kobayashi J, et al: Surgical management of children with temporal lobe epilepsy. Neurosurgery 1987;21:792–797.

9 Gonzales D, Elvidge AR: On the occurrence of epilepsy caused by astrocytoma of the cerebral hemispheres. J Neurosurg 1962;19:470–482.

10 Black P McL, Ronner SF: Cortical mapping for defining the limits of tumor resection. Neurosurgery 1987;20:914–919.

11 Penfield W, Boldrey E: Somatic motor and sensory representation in the cerebral cortex of man as studied by electrical stimulation. Brain 1937;60:389–443.

12 Gregorie EM, Goldring S: Localization of function in the excision of lesions from the sensorimotor region. J Neurosurg 1984;61:1047–1054.

13 Wada J, Rasmussen T: Intracarotid injections of sodium amytal for the lateralization of cerebral speech dominance. J Neurosurg 1960;17:266–282.

14 Berger MS, Ojemann GA, Lettich E: Neurophysiological monitoring during astrocytoma surgery. Neurosurg Clin North Am 1990;1:65–80.
15 Rostomily RC, Berger MS, Ojemann GA, et al: Postoperative deficits and functional recovery following removal of tumors involving the dominant hemisphere supplementory motor area. J Neurosurg, in press.
16 Ojemann GA, Ojemann J, Lettich E, et al: Cortical language localization in left, dominant hemisphere. J Neurosurg 1989;71:316–326.
17 Fritsch G, Hitzig E: Über die elektrische Erregbarkeit des Grosshirns. Arch Anat Physiol Wiss 1870, p 100.
18 Penfield W, Roberts L: Speech and Brain Mechanisms. Princeton, Princeton University Press, 1959.

Mitchel S. Berger, MD, Department of Neurological Surgery,
University of Washington, University Hospital, RI-20,
1959 Pacific Street, Seattle, WA 98195 (USA)

Proceedings of the Meeting of the American Society for Stereotactic and Functional Neurosurgery, Pittsburgh, Pa., June 16–19, 1991
Stereotact Funct Neurosurg 1992;58:162–167

Corticoamygdalectomy in Memory-Impaired Patients

Hyoung-Ihl Kim, André Olivier, Marilyn Jones-Gotman, David Primrose, Frederick Andermann

Montreal Neurological Institute and Hospital, and Department of Neurology and Neurosurgery, McGill University, Montreal, Que., Canada

Key Words. Epilepsy · Amygdalectomy · Memory

Abstract. Sixty-seven patients who underwent resection of the amygdala and temporal neocortex for intractable temporal lobe epilepsy were analyzed. Forty-four of them failed memory tests during the intracarotid sodium amytal procedure or showed severe impairment of contralateral material specific memory. Surgical outcome ratings were seizure-free or rare seizure, 51%; worthwhile improvement, 15%; failure, 34%. The least successful outcome was noted in the group with mandatory corticoamygdalectomy and seizure origin in the dominant hemisphere. There was no postoperative exacerbation of memory deficit, whether preoperative memory was normal or impaired. When hippocampal resection is inadvisable, corticoamygdalectomy may be considered.

The generation of seizure activity in the amygdala and hippocampus and its propagation to the temporal neocortex are critical features of temporal lobe epilepsy. Accordingly, anterior temporal resection including medial temporal structures has been known to be the most effective surgical approach [1]. However, it is not always possible to resect medial structures, especially the hippocampal formation. If hippocampal structures ipsilateral to resection cannot be compensated by the opposite side, they should not be resected, in order to avoid persisting postsurgical memory deficit [2].

We have been performing amygdalectomy under the assumption that the amygdala is a potent generator of seizure activity along with the hippocampus [3], that unilateral amygdalectomy does not aggravate the degree of memory impairment [4] and that amygdalectomy interrupts extensive connections [5]. Additionally, temporal corticectomy

1011–6125/92/0584–0162 $ 2.75/0

could eliminate epileptogenic temporal neocortex and reduce conduction of seizure activity through neocortical structures.

In this study, we examined surgical outcome in patients who underwent corticoamygdalectomy and assessed postoperative memory changes, especially in patients who failed memory tests during an intracarotid sodium amytal (ISA) procedure or who showed severe impairment of contralateral material-specific memory.

Subjects and Methods

Subjects

Sixty-seven patients were studied. Excluded were patients who had an atypical speech representation, full-scale IQ below 80, space-occupying lesions, psychiatric disturbances or age outside the range of 16–50 years.

Thirty-five patients were male and 32 female. Twenty-four patients were operated on the right and 43 on the left. Mean age at operation was 26.3 ± 9 years. Age of onset and duration from seizure onset to operation were 9.7 ± 8.2 and 16.4 ± 7.7 years, respectively. All patients have been followed up for more than 2 years.

Neuropsychological Tests

Four memory tests, two comprised of verbal material and two of designs, were performed in all patients preoperatively and 2 weeks after operation. Forty-one were reexamined 1 year after operation. Twenty-eight patients (13 right/15 left) failed memory tests during ISA procedures, and 13 showed severe memory impairment on noninvasive tests but did not undergo ISA testing. As it was mandatory to leave the hippocampus intact in these patients because of poor memory, they were considered as a mandatory group. In the remaining patients, the hippocampus was left intact because of localization of seizure discharge in neocortex or amygdala, technical difficulty during operation, particularly efficient memory or a job relying on memory; they constituted a control group.

Extent of Resections

Following removal of anterior temporal neocortex, the temporal horn was opened to expose the posterior portion of the amygdala. This structure was removed as completely as possible with an ultrasonic dissector (CUSA) under magnification, but small dorsal and medial portions of the amygdala were left to prevent injury to surrounding structures. Therefore, the resection included anterior temporal neocortex, most of the amygdala and the anterior segment of the uncus. The average size of corticectomy was 52 mm along the sylvian fissure on the right and 45 mm on the left.

Statistical Analysis

Results from the two verbal memory tests were combined into a single verbal memory score, and the same was done with the two design memory tests. These data were submitted to two-way analyses of variance, followed by post-hoc comparisons

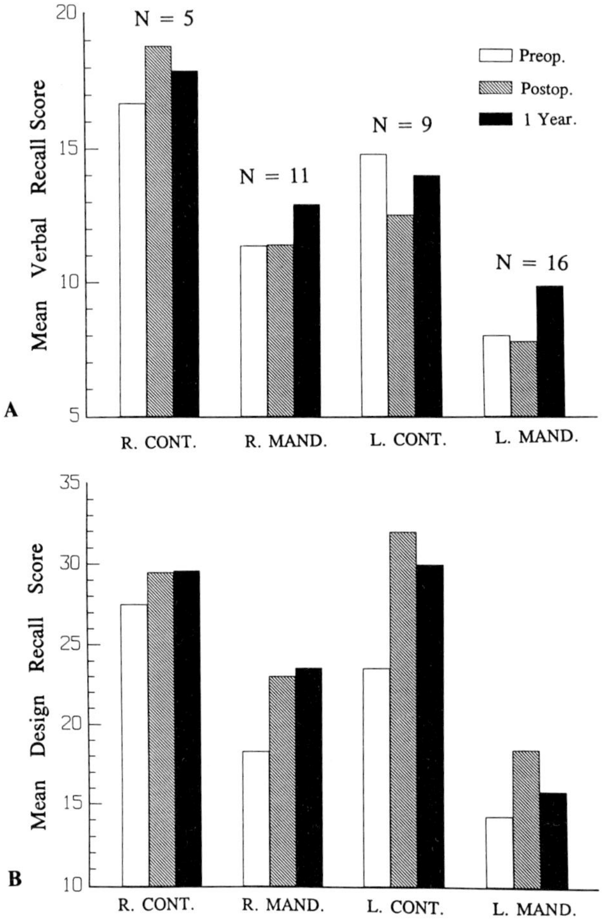

Fig. 1. Mean scores earned by the four patient groups before operation, 2 weeks postoperatively and at 1 year follow-up. CONT. = Control group; MAND. = mandatory group. **A** Combined verbal recall scores (prose passages and paired-associates). Maximum = 33. **B** Combined design recall scores (Wechsler Memory Scale designs and Rey-Osterrieth figure). Maximum = 50.

where applicable, using the Newman-Keuls test. Several seizure-related or operative variables were examined by discriminant analysis to determine which factors influenced outcome. Factors included were age of onset, duration of seizures and size of resection. Surgical outcome was classified into three categories: patients classified as A were

Table 1. Surgical outcome in four patient groups

Group	n	Outcome, %		
		A	B	C
Right control	7	43	29	29
Right mandatory	17	53	29	18
Left control	16	56	13	31
Left mandatory	27	48	4	48
Total	67	51	15	34

completely seizure-free or had fewer than 3 attacks per year; B denoted a reduction of more than 50% in the number of attacks, and C cases had lesser improvement or failure.

Results

Neuropsychological Changes

The analysis of variance on verbal memory scores revealed significant differences among the groups ($F = 14.3$, $p < 0.01$), but time of testing (preoperative, postoperative or 1 year follow-up) was not significant ($F = 1.7$) and there was no interaction ($F = 1.2$). The significant group effect was analyzed further with a Newman-Keuls comparison. This showed a deficit in the left mandatory group compared to both control groups and to the right mandatory group; also the right mandatory group had a significant deficit compared to the right control group (fig. 1A). The analysis of combined design recall showed significant differences among the groups ($F = 10.1$, $p < 0.01$) and testing times ($F = 8.1$, $p < 0.01$), but there was not a significant interaction ($F = 0.8$). Newman-Keuls comparisons again revealed a significant deficit in the left mandatory group compared to both control groups and to the right mandatory group. The time of testing analysis showed a significant improvement after surgery, present both in early postoperative tests ($p < 0.01$) and at 1 year follow-up ($p < 0.01$; fig. 1B).

Surgical Outcome

Table 1 shows the surgical results for each group. The outcome was not different between control and mandatory groups. However, the left mandatory group showed the least success. Discriminant analysis showed that the size of resection differed significantly among groups, reflecting smaller resection in the dominant hemisphere. It was not correlated statistically with the prediction of outcome. Other seizure-related variables did not significantly predict outcome.

Discussion

The amygdala has been a major target of kindling to produce epileptic activity in experimental models of epilepsy [6]. Furthermore, it has been considered a potent generator of epileptic activity in temporal lobe epilepsy [3]. Fifty-one percent of the patients in our series became seizure-free or had rare seizures, and 15% had worthwhile improvement despite sparing of the hippocampal formation. This suggests that the amygdala has an important role in temporal lobe epilepsy and that resection of hippocampus is not essential to control seizure in many patients. However, according to our previous analysis [7], better outcome can be achieved when both amygdala and hippocampus are included in the resection.

The least successful outcome was noted in the left mandatory group in our series. This was not correlated statistically with a smaller resection of left temporal lobe compared with the right. However, the preoperative neuropsychological findings showed the lowest scores in the left mandatory group. Their more severe cognitive impairment may reflect more diffuse brain damage in those patients compared to the other groups. Prognosis seems worse in patients who have both severe memory impairment and whose seizures originate in the dominant hemisphere.

There is evidence that the amygdala participates in mnemonic processing, and its resection results in memory deficits in both experimental animals [8] and humans [9]. In contrast, our results showed no permanent loss in either verbal or design memory, whether presurgical memory was normal or impaired. Some patients of the left mandatory group did show a temporary decline in verbal recall score. We suspect that this was caused by operative manipulation and resulting brain swelling rather than by the amygdalectomy itself.

In conclusion, corticoamygdalectomy is a relatively safe procedure even in memory-impaired patients, and allows the preservation of memory function. It may be considered in patients who are not candidates for hippocampal resection because they have or may be expected to develop memory deficit.

References

1 Rasmussen TB: Surgical treatment of complex partial seizures: Results, lessons, and problems. Epilepsia 1983;24(suppl 1):S65–S76.
2 Scoville WB, Milner B: Loss of recent memory after bilateral hippocampal lesion. J Neurol Neurosurg Psychiatry 1957;20:11–21.
3 Feindel W, Penfield W: Localization of discharge in temporal lobe automatism. Arch Neurol Psychiatry 1954;72:605–630.
4 Milner B: Memory and the medial temporal regions of the brain; in Pribram KH, Broadbent DE (eds): Biology of Memory. New York, Academic Press, 1970, pp 29–50.
5 de Olmos JS: Amygdala; in Paxinos G (ed): The Human Nervous System. New York, Academic Press, 1990, pp 583–710.
6 Racine RJ: Kindling: The first decade. Neurosurgery 1978;3:234–252.
7 Olivier A: Risk and benefit in the surgery of epilepsy: Complication and positive results on seizure tendences and intellectual function. Acta Neurol Scand Suppl 1988;117:114–121.
8 Mishkin M: Memory in monkeys severely impaired by combined but not by separate removal of amygdala and hippocampus. Nature 1978;273:297–298.
9 Andersen R: Cognitive changes after amygdalectomy. Neuropsychologia 1978;16: 439–451.

H.-I. Kim, MD, Department of Neurosurgery, Chonbuk National University Hospital, Chonju 560-180 (Republic of Korea)

Proceedings of the Meeting of the American Society for Stereotactic and Functional Neurosurgery, Pittsburgh, Pa., June 16–19, 1991
Stereotact Funct Neurosurg 1992;58:168–171

Surgery of Central Sensory Motor and Dorsolateral Frontal Lobe Seizures

M.F. Levesque, W.W. Sutherling, P.H. Crandall
Division of Neurosurgery and Department of Neurology,
UCLA School of Medicine, Los Angeles, Calif., USA

Key Words. Epilepsy surgery · Frontal lobe epilepsy · Sensory motor cortex · Dorsolateral frontal lobe · Epilepsy

Abstract. Ten patients who presented with dorsolateral or frontocentral seizures were studied with chronic subdural grid electrodes. Cortical mapping, sensory-evoked potentials and chronic electrocorticography were obtained for each patient. Seizures were classified as focal, regional or dipolar. At the time of explantation, a selective functional corticectomy was performed. Surgical outcome is presented at a mean follow-up of 36 months. Two patients are seizure-free and 7 patients had a significant reduction in seizure frequency. One patient had no change in seizure pattern. Dorsolateral frontal lobe seizures have a focal functional anatomy and can be surgically treated by selective cortectomy.

Frontal lobe epilepsy remains a surgical challenge because of the variability of clinical and electrographic presentations [1]. Despite wide frontal resections, the surgical outcome has remained suboptimal and poorer than temporal lobe resection for temporo-limbic epilepsy. New methods to determine whether frontal lobe seizures can have focal functional anatomy were prospectively analyzed in patients who presented with dorsolateral frontal central epilepsies [2]. Because of their unique semiology or previous stereotactic depth electrode studies indicating a neocortical dorsolateral frontal onset, high-resolution mapping of cortical function and seizure patterns were obtained. This was followed by selective corticectomy guided by the ictal onset and normal anatomy as determined by subdural grid studies. We present the surgical results of this subgroup of patients [3].

1011–6125/92/0584–0168 $ 2.75/0

Table 1. Characteristics of the patients

Patient	Age years	Sex	Seizure duration years	Seizure type	Resection	Outcome
1	28	M	20	S, C, G	L prefrontal	III
2	37	M	4	S, C, G	L premotor	II
3	22	F	19	S	R prefrontal	I
4	47	M	7	S, C	L prefrontal	III
5	29	M	16	S, G	R frontocentral	II
6	33	M	16	S, G	R frontocentral	II
7	12	M	9	S, C, G	L prefrontal	I
8	14	M	7	S, C	R frontocentral	I
9	25	F	20	S, C	L frontocentral	IV
10	32	M	10	S, G	L frontocentral	II

M = Male; F = female; L = left; R = right; S = simple complex; C = complex; G = generalized. I–IV see text.

Clinical Material and Methods

Ten patients were included in this study. Each patient presented with medically intractable seizures and had semiologies suggesting either focal frontal or frontal central origin. All patients underwent noninvasive studies, including video telemetry monitoring, MRI and PET studies. They also underwent standard neuropsychometric testing and intracarotid Amytal testing.

Surgical Procedure

Subdural grids were implanted after a wide craniotomy was performed, with the patient under general anesthesia. The area covered varied according the semiology but consistently covered the dorsolateral frontal lobe and central cortex. Postoperatively, each patient underwent a battery of standard cortical stimulation and evoked potential studies, followed by seizure recordings and continuous 24-hour telemetry monitoring. Seizure onset was classified according to the initial changes on electrocorticographic recording as focal, regional or dipolar. Three weeks after initial implantation, the craniotomy was reopened under local or general anesthesia. Results of the cortical mapping were correlated in 2 patients with bipolar stimulation. The zone of seizure origin was determined and a resection was performed, using microsurgical techniques to preserve ascending vessels. Postoperatively, the patients underwent standard MRI and psychometric studies. Follow-up at a mean of 36 months is presented and classified as follows: class I, seizure-free: class II, reduction by at least 80% in seizure frequency: class III, reduction by at least 50% in seizure frequency, and class IV, less than 50% reduction in seizure frequency.

Results

Patient age varied from 12 to 47 years with a mean age of 27 years (table 1). There were 8 males and 2 females. Seizure duration varied from 4 to 20 years with a mean duration of 12 years. Seizure semiology consisted of simple partial seizures, which became either complex or generalized in 9 patients. Neuroimaging studies showed either normal anatomy or localized atrophy. PET was read as either normal or with subtle lateralized hypometabolism. Scalp EEGs showed ictal changes which were lateralized in the frontal lobe in 8 cases. Normal functional anatomy was mapped in all patients, and included sensory and motor cortex as well as language sensitive sites on the dominant hemisphere. Seizure onset was defined as focal in 4 patients, regional in 3 and dipolar in 3. There were 6 left-sided resections and 4 right-sided. Resections involved the motor or prefrontal cortex in 5 patients and the frontal central cortex in 5 patients. At a mean follow-up of 36 months, 3 patients were seizure-free, 4 had at least an 80% reduction in seizure frequency, 3 had a reduction of at least 50%, and 1 patient had no change in seizure frequency.

Discussion

Frontal lobe epilepsy can present with a wide variety of ictal and electrographic onsets. Classification of frontal lobe epilepsy can be attempted based on the neuroanatomy of the frontal lobe. All of our patients presented with simple partial seizures, suggesting a focal onset within the central cortex or prefrontal cortex with a rapid propagation to the central sensory motor cortex. These patients showed no evidence of a structural mass lesion according to their neuroimaging studies. Seizure recording established a focal onset in 4 patients and regional onset in 3. In addition, focality was achieved by computerized analysis of ictal changes as a dipolar onset, somewhat similar to the dipole produced by sensory-evoked potentials. Resection was guided by the boundaries defined by the ictal onset without attempting to include the zone of interictal abnormalities or propagation pattern.

Our relatively short follow-up appeared to support the concept of focal epileptogenicity in this group of patients. Rasmussen [4] previously pointed out in a series of 40 patients with frontal lobe epilepsy who became seizure-free after resection that refinement and quantification of epileptiform changes are essential to improve satisfactory definition of the resection boundaries. Our study demonstrated that patients with dorsolateral frontal lobe seizured can have focal functional anatomy and a surgical resection can produce a satisfactory outcome.

References

1 Bancaud J, Talairach J, et al: La stéréo-éléctroencéphalographie dans l'épiléspsie. Paris, Masson, 1965.
2 Sutherling WW, Risinger MW, et al: Focal functional anatomy of dorsolateral frontocentral seizures. Neurosurgery 1990;40:87–99.
3 Levesque MF, Sutherling WW: Surgical exploration and treatment of frontal lobe epilepsies. J Neurosurgery, submitted.
4 Rasmussen T: Characteristics of a pure culture of frontal lobe epilepsy. Epilepsia 1983;24:482–493.

M.F. Levesque, MD, Division of Neurosurgery and Department of Neurology, UCLA School of Medicine, 760 Westwood Plaza, Los Angeles, CA 90024 (USA)

Proceedings of the Meeting of the American Society for Stereotactic and Functional Neurosurgery, Pittsburgh, Pa., June 16–19, 1991
Stereotact Funct Neurosurg 1992;58:172–177

Surgical Outcome in Computer-Assisted Stereotactic Resection of Intra-Axial Cerebral Lesions for Partial Epilepsy

Nayef R.F. Al-Rodhan[a], *Patrick J. Kelly*[a], *Gregory D. Cascino*[b], *Frank W. Sharbrough*[b]

Departments of [a] Neurosurgery and [b] Neurology, Mayo Clinic and Mayo Graduate School of Medicine, Rochester, Minn., USA

Key Words. Partial epilepsy · Cortical resection · Stereotactic lesion resection · Surgical management · Eloquent cortex

Abstract. A retrospective analysis was performed in 30 patients who underwent computer-assisted stereotactic resection of intra-axial mass lesions with intractable partial epilepsy. Mean follow-up was 4.1 years (2–5.5), mean age 21 years (3–45) and mean duration of seizures 8.4 years (1–26). Pathology consisted of vascular malformations in 11, glial neoplasms in 11, cortical dysplasia in 4 and gliosis in 3, and no diagnostic abnormality was found in 2 patients. The location of the lesions in some cases may have precluded a standard craniotomy and cortical resection, e.g. precentral gyrus (5), postcentral gyrus (5) and deep-seated left posterior temporal region (4). Operative morbidity involved 3 patients who developed motor or language deficits. Four patients were lost to follow-up. Thirteen patients out of 26 (50%) were class I, 3 (12%) were class II, 4 (15%) were class III and 6 (23%) were class IV. These findings suggest that stereotactic lesion resection in selected cases (e.g. where lesions are located in eloquent brain regions) can be useful in providing a histological diagnosis of the epileptogenic foci and result in a favorable reduction in seizure activity without the need for a standard cortical resection.

While it is generally accepted that cortical resection in patients with intractable seizures is an effective mode of therapy [1, 2], results of surgical resection of epileptogenic lesions have been less clear [3–5]. In this brief paper, we present out technique and follow-up with 30 computer-assisted stereotactic lesion resections of intra-axial cerebral le-

1011–6125/92/0584–0172 $ 2.75/0

a 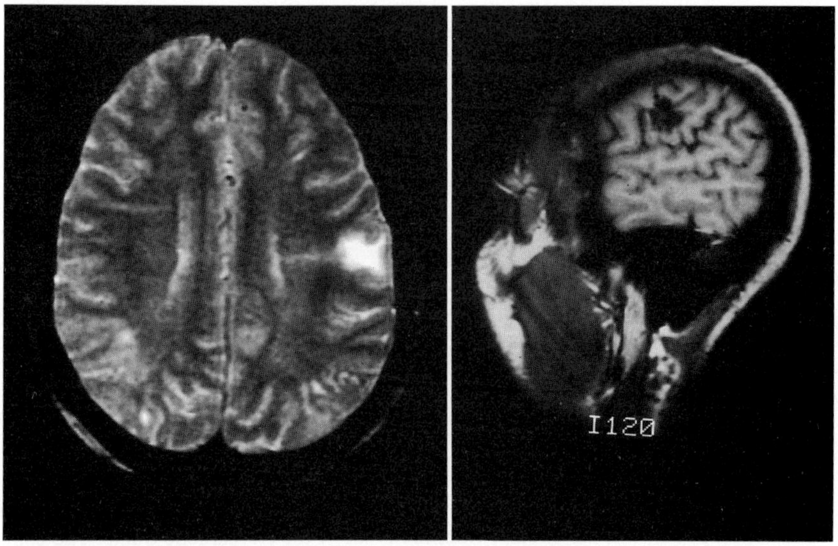 b

Fig. 1. MR images of the brain of a patient with medically refractory seizures. **a** Lesion in the posterior frontal region. **b** Postoperative defect following the resection of an AVM.

sions for intractable seizures. The advantages of this stereotactic method in resecting intra-axial lesions involving functional or eloquent cortex are outlined.

Clinical Material and Methods

Between 1984 and 1988, 30 patients (25 male, 5 female; mean age 25 years) with intractable epilepsy (mean duration of seizures 8.4 years) underwent computer-assisted stereotactic lesion resection at the Mayo Clinic. Patients were considered refractory to medical therapy if the seizures were not controlled by maximally tolerated monotherapy or combination antiepileptic therapy that consisted of phenytoin, carbamazepine, phenobarbital and primidone.

Modes of presentation of these patients were: 20 patients had complex partial seizures; 13 had simple partial seizures; 12 had secondary generalized tonic-clonic seizures, and 15 had multiple types of seizures. All patients underwent scalp-recorded awake and sleep EEG, and CT or MRI, or both. Prolonged video EEG monitoring was performed in 18 of the 30 patients and electrocorticography (ECOG) was performed in 16. Preoperative imaging studies revealed a structural abnormality in all patients

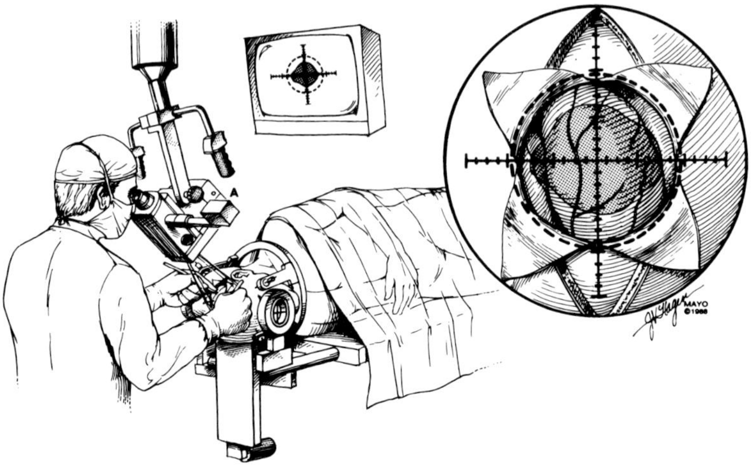

Fig. 2. Diagram of method for stereotactic resection of superficial intra-axial brain lesions. The position of the circular trephine is set by the stereotactic frame. The computer slices the tumor volume defined by CT and MRI with respect to the surgical viewline and position of the circular trephine, and displays the tumor slice image within a circle that represents the position and configuration of the trephine. This scaled information is displayed on a video monitor and also projected into a 'heads-up' display unit on the operating microscope. The surgeon positions the microscope so that the image of the trephine in the heads-up display unit is superimposed over the actual trephine in the surgical field. The configuration of the CT- and MRI-defined tumor slices is also superimposed on the surgical field in order to indicate the location, configuration and extent of the subcortical lesion at each successive depth level. (Reprinted with permission from Mayo Clin Proc 1988;63:1186–1198.)

(fig. 1). The location of the structural abnormality correlated well with both the clinical and EEG data. The awake and sleep EEG studies were performed using the standard placement of 10–20 electrodes, with elective placement of additional electrodes as needed. Hyperventilation and photic stimulation were used as activation procedures.

Computer-assisted stereotactic resections of intra-axial lesions are performed in three phases: data base acquisition, treatment planning and the interactive procedure. The details of our technique have been described elsewhere [6]. In brief, this involves a replaceable CT- and MRI-compatible stereotactic head frame. After the application of the head frame, the patient undergoes stereotactic CT, MRI and digital angiographic examination. After data acquisition, the stereotactic surgical approach to the lesion is then planned at the computer console. The technical aspects of the surgical procedure (fig. 2) will depend on whether the lesion is located superficially or deep [6].

Postoperative seizure frequency was determined through correspondence, medical records and by directly contacting patients. Seizure outcome was classified accord-

Table 1. Surgical outcome in 30 patients who underwent stereotactic lesion resection for partial epilepsy (mean follow-up 4.1 years)

Class	n	Histological findings				
		GN	VM	CD	G	NDA
I	13[a]	8	4	1	1	
II	3		2		1	
III	4		1	1		2
IV	6	3	2	1		
Lost to follow-up	4		2	1	1	

[a] An astrocytoma and cortical dysplasia were present in 1 specimen.
GN = Glial neoplasm; VM = vascular malformation; G = gliosis; CD = cortical dysplasia; NDA = no diagnostic abnormality.

ing to the alteration in seizure activity postoperatively compared to the preoperative level: class I = seizure-free after surgery, auras only or a single seizure episode; class II = rare seizure activity postoperatively (less than 3 seizure episodes per year); class III = marked reduction in seizure activity postoperatively (≥90% reduction in seizures), and class IV = moderate or no reduction seizure in activity (<90% reduction in seizures).

Results

Sixteen patients had lesions in eloquent cortex: parietal lobe (including postcentral gyrus; n = 6); precentral gyrus (n = 4); left mesial posterior temporal lobe (n = 3); temporoparietal region (n = 1); fronto-operculum (language dominant hemisphere; n = 1), and occipital lobe (n = 1).

Complications involved 3 patients: 1 patient developed a transient right upper monoparesis after the resection of a left parietal arteriovenous malformation (AVM). This eventually resolved. The second patient developed a reduction in rapid alternating movement in his left hand after the resection of a lesion (pathology nondiagnostic) from the right motor cortex. The third patient developed transient anomic dysphasia after the resection of an AVM from the left mesial temporal cortex. This eventually resolved. No other complications were observed.

The long-term outcome of these patients (mean follow-up 4.1 years) showed: class I, 13 patients (50%); class II, 3 patients (12%); class III, 4 patients (15%), and class IV, 6 patients (23%; table 1).

Discussion

This study indicates that stereotactic excision of an epileptogenic lesion can result in significant reduction in seizure activity in carefully selected patients even when anticonvulsant therapy is discontinued. A preliminary report with a shorter follow-up was published previously [4].

The localization of the lesion or its histological type did not statistically influence the class of postoperative seizure control. Intraoperative mapping of cortical function may have prevented the morbidity associated with resection of lesions in eloquent cortex. The effect of the extent of resection on outcome could not be determined since the neuroradiologic abnormality was completely resected in all patients.

While this technique is not meant to be a replacement for detailed mapping studies and standard cortical resections, nevertheless it has certain advantages. The advantages of this stereotactic technique include the low surgical morbidity with a smaller cranial opening, minimal invasiveness and shorter hospital stay. A significant number of patients will derive benefit from simply removing the intracranial lesion associated with the seizures. There may be some patients within this group who may ultimately require invasive monitoring and more extensive cortical resection. There is no reason why this small percentage of patients cannot undergo these more extensive procedures at a later date if seizure control is suboptimal. However, in important intracranial locations, a more extensive cortical resection may not be advisable anyway.

In conclusion, stereotactic resection of selected cortical and subcortical lesions is a reasonable 'first step' in the management of focal epilepsy.

References

1 Dreifuss FE: Goals of surgery for epilepsy; in Engel J Jr (ed): Surgical Treatment of the Epilepsies. New York, Raven Press, 1987, pp 31–49.
2 Engel J Jr: Alternate treatment; in Engel J Jr (ed): Seizures and Epilepsy. Philadelphia, Davis, 1989, pp 443–474.
3 Spencer DD, Spencer SS, Mattson RH, et al: Intracerebral masses in patients with intractable partial epilepsy. Neurology 1984;34:432–436.
4 Cascino GD, Kelly PJ, Hirschorn KA, et al: Stereotactic resection of intra-axial cerebral lesions in partial epilepsy. Mayo Clin Proc 1990;65:1053–1060.
5 Goldring S, Rich K, Picker S: Experience with gliomas in patients presenting with a chronic seizure disorder; in Little JR (ed): Clinical Neurosurgery. Baltimore, Williams & Wilkins, 1986, vol 33, pp 15–42.
6 Kelly PJ: Tumor Stereotaxis. Philadelphia, Saunders, 1991.

Nayef Al-Rodhan, MD, PhD, Department of Neurosurgery, Mayo Clinic,
Rochester, MN 55905 (USA)

Proceedings of the Meeting of the American Society for Stereotactic and Functional Neurosurgery, Pittsburgh, Pa., June 16–19, 1991
Stereotact Funct Neurosurg 1992;58:178

Focal Encephalitis as an Etiology of Temporal Lobe Epilepsy

N.M. Barbaro, T.J. Rosenbaum, K.D. Laxer
Department of Neurosurgery, UCSF, San Francisco, Calif., USA

In 1958, Rasmussen described a syndrome of chronic focal encephalitis which included progressive hemiparesis, focal hemispheric atrophy and intractable seizures, most commonly epilepsia partialis continua. Pathological evaluation of tissue obtained from these patients revealed perivascular lymphocytic cuffing, microglial nodules, and spongy degeneration. In the original series of 27 patients, 25 developed progressive neurological deficits involving much of one hemisphere. We have found similar pathological findings in 8 patients undergoing temporal lobectomy for medically refractory complex partial seizures. These 8 cases were found among 160 patients operated at two epilepsy centers. There were no differences in the past medical histories, seizure types, family histories, radiological studies or telemetry findings between these cases and the other patients who underwent temporal lobectomies. These patients did have a significantly later seizure onset (12.9 vs. 9.9 years) and came to surgery at an earlier average age (22.1 vs. 25.4 years) than patients with other pathological findings. Electrocorticography revealed widespread interictal epileptiform activity which usually persisted following resection of the anterior temporal lobe. With follow-up ranging from 1 to 6 years, only 1 patient has been seizure-free following temporal lobectomy compared with 65% of the other patients. Two of these patients developed progressive neurological deterioration including focal motor seizures, while the others have had stable neurological examinations. Chronic focal encephalitis may present as a focal pathological disorder in the temporal lobe, and may be a cause of medically refractory seizures. Although these 8 patients represent only 4% of the patients who underwent temporal lobectomy, they comprise approximately 25% of the cases which did not show substantial postoperative improvement in seizure frequency. Unfortunately, there have been no clinical or radiographic features with which to diagnose these cases preoperatively. Longer follow-up of these patients is required before their overall prognosis is known.

1011–6125/92/0584–0178 $ 2.75/0

Proceedings of the Meeting of the American Society for Stereotactic and Functional Neurosurgery, Pittsburgh, Pa., June 16–19, 1991
Stereotact Funct Neurosurg 1992;58:179–188

Use of the Callosal Grid System for the Preoperative Identification of the Central Sulcus

R.M. Lehman, A. Olivier, J.-J. Moreau, D. Tampieri, C. Henri
Montreal Neurological Hospital and Institute, Montreal, Que., Canada

Key Words. Stereotactic surgery · Midcallosal grid system · Central sulcus

Abstract. The callosal grid system based on modern imaging techniques facilitates the identification of the central sulcus by its relationship to the midcallosal plane. Imaging with or without the stereotactic frame allows precise localization of various anatomic sites, which can be compartmentalized within subdivisions of the grid system. The information gained permits accurate preoperative planning and intraoperative recognition of the central sulcus and adjacent neurovascular structures.

The central sulcus is a landmark of paramount importance both for open craniotomy and stereotactic procedures. Its identification, however, remains difficult. Extensive anatomic and angiographic work has been done to determine the course and variable branching patterns of the middle cerebral artery [1–13]. Localization of the central sulcus by angiography has been described by Ring and Waddington [14] and Szikla et al. [12]. Stereoscopic arteriovenous digital subtraction angiography (DSA) has facilitated this approach. MRI can be superimposed on the DSA and the position of the central sulcus can be studied [15, 16]. To further clarify the identification of the central sulcus, we have made use of an original callosal grid system, which is established by a series of lines and planes based on the corpus callosum, taken as the basic landmark [15–18]. Initial work indicated the close relationship of one of these lines to the central region.

1011–6125/92/0584–0179 $ 2.75/0

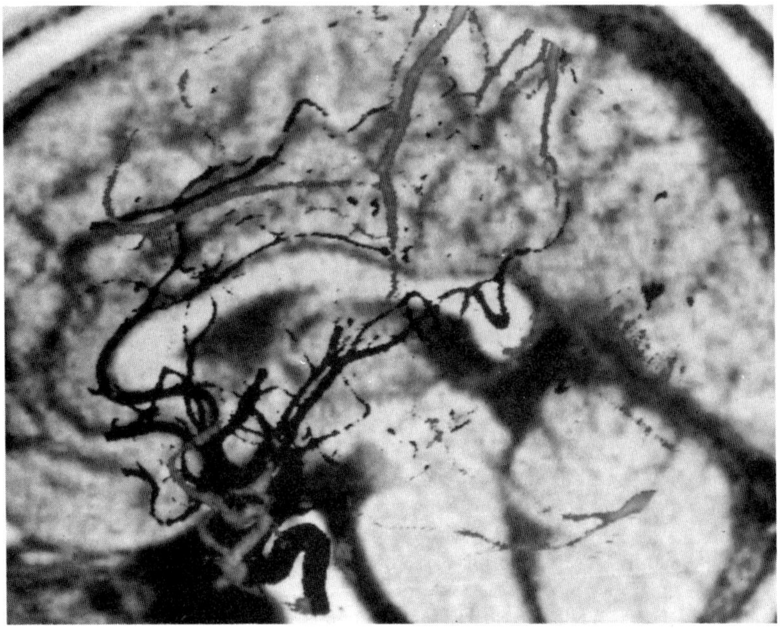

Fig. 1. Identification of corpus callosum on superimposed DSA and MRI.

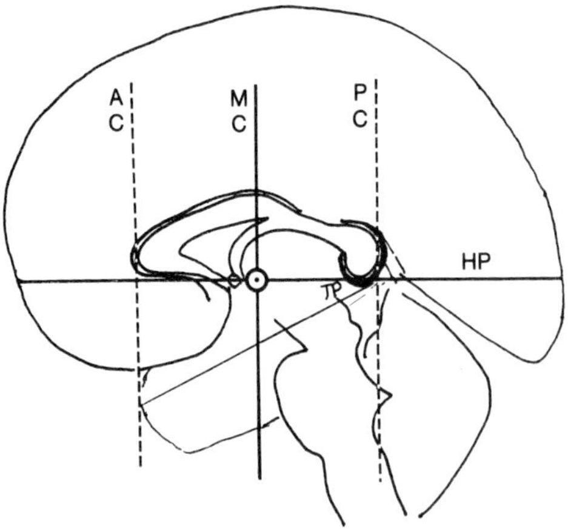

Fig. 2. Callosal grid system.

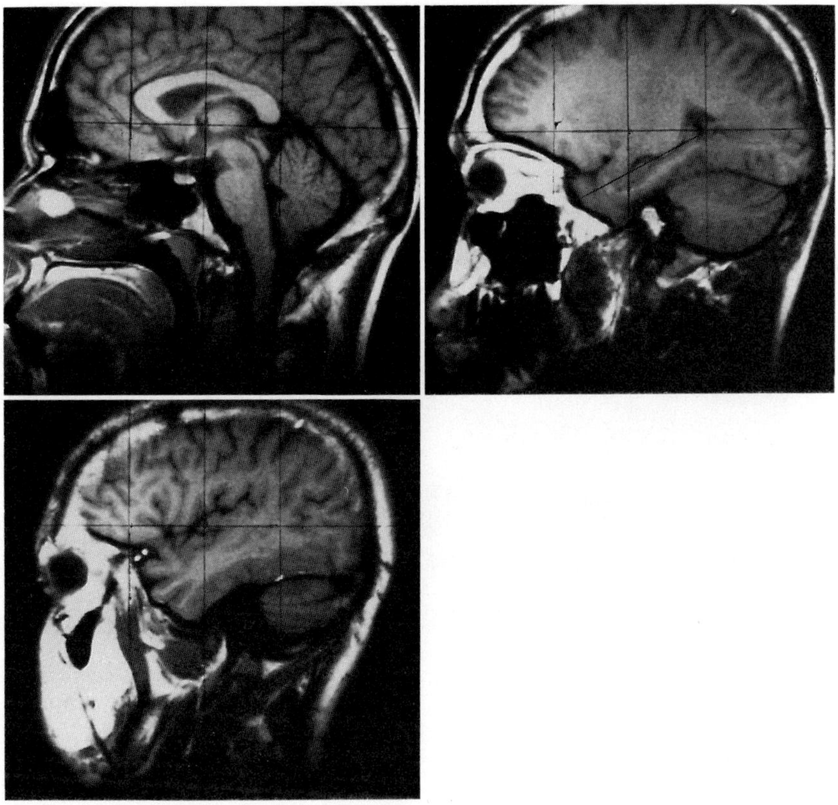

a b c

Fig. 3. MR images. **a** Midsagittal. **b** 'Limbic' parasagittal. **c** 'Cortical' parasagittal. Note: MC in relation to inferior central sulcus.

Materials and Methods

The corpus callosum can be identified indirectly on the arteriovenous DSA and directly on the midsagittal MRI (fig. 1). A horizontal plane (HP) is constructed through the inferior border of the genu and splenium of the corpus callosum. Three vertical planes perpendicular to HP are created: an anterior callosal plane (AC), tangential to the anterior border of the genu, a posterior callosal plane (PC), tangential to the posterior border of the splenium, and a midcallosal plane (MC) which corresponds to the midpoint between AC and PC (fig. 2).

Using this callosal grid system, the DSA and MR images of 100 consecutive cases were analyzed by films (fig. 3, 4) and three-dimensional computer terminal [19–21]

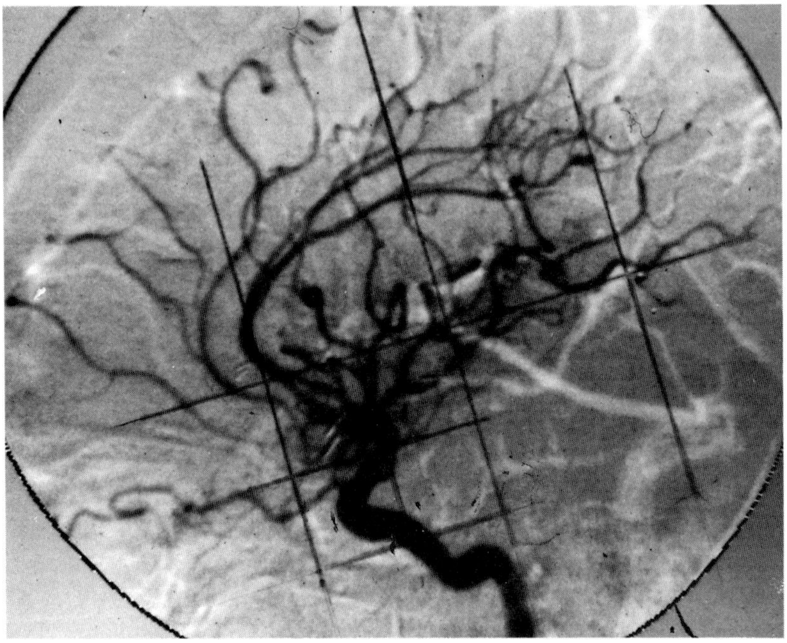

Fig. 4. DSA. Note: relationship MC to central artery.

(fig. 5). The last 40 cases were studied in detail as to the relationship not only of the central artery, but the entire central sulcus, amygdala, insula and temporal plane within the grid system. The length of the corpus callosum, the entire brain length, and the anterior and posterior pole lengths created by the vertical planes were also recorded. The simultaneous viewing of the DSA and MRI on the stereo computer allowed cross-correlation of stereotactic points by a cursor interactive between the modalities of imaging.

Additionally, 10 cadaver brains were dissected after the intracranial vessels were perfused with latex. In 3 brains a mixture of barium sulfate and latex was used to allow CT and MR imaging before dissection. Of interest was the finding of a major central artery from a branch of the inferior division (M2) of the middle cerebral artery in 4 of the 20 hemispheres. The brain specimens were further evaluated by a callosal grid system created by a solid plastic template placed against the mesial side of the hemisphere with holes parallel and perpendicular in rows to allow probes to be passed through the brain in the callosal grid planes. As the probes pierced the cortex on the lateral surface, the relationship of the projected callosal planes could be directly determined in relation to the central artery and sulcus, as well as adjacent sulci and arteries. The brain was then sectioned along these callosal planes both horizontally and vertically, and the

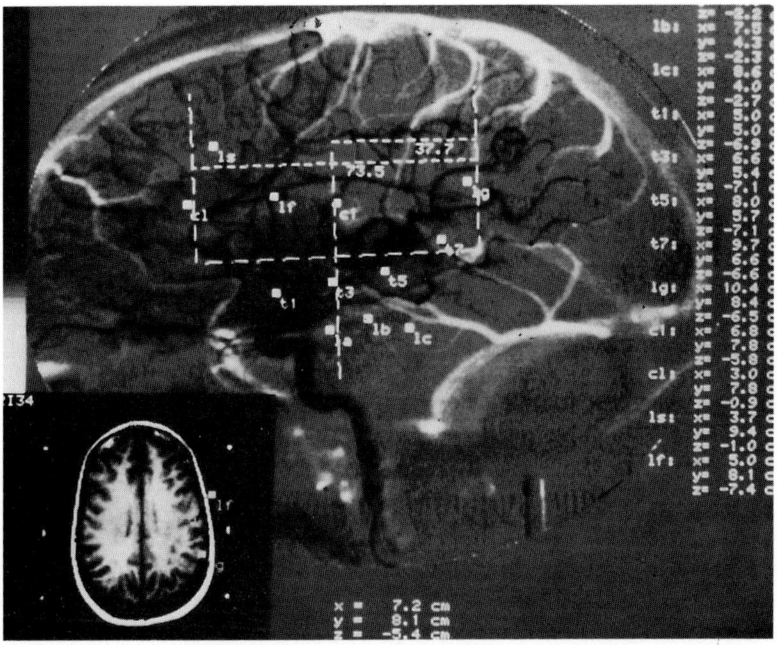

Fig. 5. Three-dimensional computer combined DSA and MRI. Note: cursor on DSA on MC at C1 with cursor on MRI in central sulcus.

cortical and subcortical structures revealed in each plane were noted. Regional gyri and sulci, projection fibers and subcortical structures could be compartmentalized using the grid system based on their location within the vertical and horizontal grid planes.

Results

MC intersects the central sulcus inferiorly at a point where the central artery enters the central sulcus in 95% of clinical cases, with a variation in 5% of cases of 3–7 mm (n = 100). The mean deviation of the inferior central sulcus was 0.3 ± 1.2 mm posterior to MC, which was verified by cadaver brain dissection with the callosal grid probes.

Table 1. Mean positions of anatomic sites within the grid system (n = 100)

Anatomic site	Position
1. CI (central sulcus, inferior point)	0.3 mm posterior to PC
2. CS (superior central sulcus, midsagittal)	4.0 mm anterior to PC
3. CMS (ascending ramus callosal marginal sulcus)	6.2 mm posterior to PC
4. Angle CI (inferior central sulcus with HP)	76.1 °
5. Angle TP (temporal plane)	28 °
6. CC length (corpus callosum)	74.4 mm
7. WB length (whole brain)	163.4 mm
8. AP length (anterior pole to AC)	36.7 mm
9. PP length (posterior pole to PC)	52.3 mm

The statistical analysis of location of the remaining anatomic sites within the grid system is compiled in table 1. The superior extension of the central sulcus at the midline (CS) was a mean of 4.0 mm anterior to PC, and the angle of the central sulcus inferior to the plane (HP) was a mean of 76 °. The course of the central sulcus between the inferior point CI, where the central artery enters the central sulcus (MC intersection), and CS, where the central sulcus reaches the midline in relation to PC, was traced by template over the MR images (fig. 3–5). Correlation of intermediate points along the central sulcus was difficult because of variation in the parasagittal sulcus on MRI. The angle of the temporal plane with the junction of HP-PC was a mean of 28 °. The mean length of the corpus callosum recorded was 74.4 mm, and of the whole brain, 163.4 mm.

Discussion

We owe the technique of orthogonal teleoangiography and stereoscopic visualization for the localization of cortical structures to Szikla and Talairach [13, 21, 22]. Their work was in part based on Duret's study [3], which revealed that the course of the cortical arteries was determined by the growth and formation of the gyri. The foldings of the brain cause the arteries to enter and leave the sulci in order to pass from one gyrus to the next. These bends and loops create a fairly typical recurrent pattern from patient to patient and delineate the sulci. By outlining the anterior and posterior commissures with ventriculography, they used these consistent deep structures to establish a grid system that allowed the integration of angiography and ventriculography for the stereotactic localization of any intracerebral structure. The lower extent of the central sulcus and artery falls between the anterior and posterior commissures. This intercommissural length formed the basis of the unit measurement for their grid system [23, 24]. The localization of the central area within this grid was further supported by electrophysiologic data in patients [11].

Recently Steinmetz et al. [25], using real-time cinematographic display of MR images in 40 hemispheres, evaluated the anatomic variability of the inferior central, precentral and postcentral sulci. Their findings revealed no right-left asymmetries for the precentral or central sulci, although the inferior postcentral sulcus tended to be located more posteriorly on the left. More important, they found a 1.5- to 2-cm variation zone of the precentral, central and postcentral sulci in the anterior-posterior axis, using the Talairach proportional grid system based on the anterior-posterior commissural line. There was minimal overlap between the sulcal zones. Moreoever, Brierley and Beck [26] found anatomic variation of diencephalic structures posterior to the posterior commissure and unrelated to the anterior-posterior commissure length.

It has been the technique at the Montreal Neurological Institute (MNI) to view angiograms in stereoscopic fashion since 1947, thus allowing better visualization of the exact course of each vessel and its branches. One of us (AO), in his preoperative anatomic planning, had noted the consistent relationship of the central artery and sulcus with the corpus callosum [17, 18]. MRI of the corpus callosum provided a more readily identifiable intracerebral landmark, which provided a more suitable basis for a grid system based on series of horizontal and vertical planes outlined by the genu and splenium. The vertical MC intersects laterally the point where the central artery enters the inferior central sulcus in a consistent and reliable manner. The remainder of the central sulcus can be identified and compartmentalized between the vertical planes MC and PC. Superiorly, the MC crosses the precentral sulcus. The works of Steinmetz et al. [25], Berger et al. [27] and more recently Ono et al. [28] outlined the high variability which makes these structures difficult to identify from one clinical case to the next. As a consequence, we think that the identification of the inferior central point, where the central artery enters the central sulcus, simplifies the localization of the central area. Imaging in the HP of the corpus callosum permits transfer of anatomic sites from DSA, MRI and even PET scans, and facilitates the recognition of the central sulcus in all these modalities. Intraoperative functional mapping has consistently confirmed our preoperative anatomic findings. The latter allows intraoperative recognition of anatomic relationships. Further, stereoencephalographic anatomic and electrophysiologic data can be combined with electrocorticographic data within the grid system on the MNI brain map. In addition, the grid system can be transferred to anatomic maps, and the electrophysiologic data superimposed for integrated display with DSA or MRI.

The consistent relationship of the inferior central point, where the central artery enters the central sulcus, to MC has some phylogenetic basis. The work of Pandya and Rosene [29], using radioactive amino acids injected into the cerebral cortex in rhesus monkeys, revealed that the motor fibers from M1 and M2 cross in the rostral half of the corpus callosum just in front of the midpoint, and the sensory fibers of S1 and S2 cross in the caudal half just behind the midpoint of the corpus callosum. It is, therefore, not surprising that this relationship of the inferior central sulcus to MC would be so consistent.

References

1 Beevor CE: The cerebral arterial supply. Brain 1907;30:403–425.
2 Serrats F, Vlahovitch B, Parker SA: The arteriographic pattern of the insula: Its normal appearance and variation in cases of tumor of the cerebral hemispheres. J Neurol Neurosurg Psychiatry 1968;31:379–390.
3 Duret H: Recherches anatomiques sur la circulation de l'encéphale. Arch Psychol Norm Pathol 1874, ser 2, pp 60–91/316–353/646–693/919–957.
4 Foix C, Levy M: Les ramolissements sylviens. Rev Neurol 1927;2:1–51.
5 Gibo H, Carver C, Rhoton A: Microsurgical anatomy of the middle cerebral artery. J Neurosurg 1981;54:151–169.
6 Jain KK: Some observations on the anatomy of the middle cerebral artery. Can J Surg 1964;7:134–139.
7 Krayenbuhl H, Yasargil MG: Radiological anatomy and topography of cerebral arteries; in Vinken PJ, Bruyn GW (eds): Vascular Diseases of the Nervous System. Handbook of Clinical Neurology. Amsterdam, North-Holland, 1972, vol 2, part 1, pp 82–86.

8 Michotey P, Moscow N, Salamon G: Anatomy of the cortical branches of the middle cerebral artery; in Newton TH, Potts DG (eds): Radiology of Skull and Brain: Angiography. St. Louis, Mosby, 1974, vol 2, pp 1471–1478.
9 Moniz E, Dias A, Lima A: La radio-artériographie et la topographie cranio-encéphalique. J Radiol 1928;12:72–82.
10 Stephens RB, Stilwell DL: Arteries and Veins of the Human Brain. Springfield, Thomas, 1969.
11 Szikla G, Talairach J: Coordinates of the rolandic sulcus and topography of cortical and subcortical motor responses to low frequency stimulation in a proportional stereotaxic system. Confin Neurol 1965;26:471–475.
12 Szikla G, Bouvier G, Hori T, Petrov V: Angiography of the Human Brain Cortex. Atlas of Vascular Patterns and Stereotactic Cortical Localization. Berlin, Springer, 1977.
13 Vlahovitch B, Frerebeau P, Kunher A, Billet M, Gros C: Etude des lignes supra- et infra-insulaires dans l'angiographie carotidienne normale et pathologique. Neurochirugie 1970;16:127–138.
14 Ring BA, Waddington MM: Angiographic identification of the motor strip. J Neurosurg 1967;26:249–254.
15 Olivier A, Peters T, Clark J, Marchand G, Mawko G, Bertrand G, Vanier M, Ethier R, Tyler J, De Lotbinière A: Intégration de l'angiographie numérique de la résonance magnétique, de la tomodensitométrie et de la tomographie par émission de positrons en stéréotaxie. Rev Electroencephalogr Neurophysiol Clin 1987; 17:25–43.
16 Peters I, Clark J, Olivier A, et al: Integrated stereotaxic imaging with CT, MRI and digital subtraction angiography. Radiology 1986;161:821–826.
17 Olivier A: Extratemporal resections in the surgical treatment of epilepsy; in Spencer S, Spencer D (eds): Surgery for Epilepsy. New York, Blackwell, 1991, pp 150–167.
18 Olivier A, De Lotbinière A: Stereotactic techniques in epilepsy. Neurosurgery 1987;2:257–285.
19 Olivier A, Marchand E, Peters T, Tyler J: Depth electrode implantation at the Montreal Neurological Institute & Hospital; in Engel J (ed): Surgical Treatment of the Epilepsies. New York, Raven Press, 1987, pp 595–601.
20 Olivier A, Peters T, Bertrand G: Stereotaxic system and apparatus for use with MRI, CT, and DSA. Appl Neurophysiol 1985;48:94–96.
21 Peters T, Henri C, Pike B, Clarke J, Collins L, Olivier A: Integration of stereoscopic DSA with three-dimensional imgage reconstruction for stereotactic planning. Stereotact Funct Neurosurg 1990;54/55:471–476.
22 Talairach J, David M, Tournoux P, Corredor H, Kvasina T. Atlas d'anatomie stéréotaxique des noyaux gris centraux. Paris, Masson, 1957.
23 Talairach J, Szikla G: Atlas of Stereotaxic Anatomy of the Telencephalon: Anatomo-Radiological Studies. Paris, Masson, 1967.
24 Talairach J, Tournoux P: Co-Planar Stereotaxic Atlas of the Human Brain. New York, Thieme, 1988.
25 Steinmetz H, Furst G, Freund HJ: Variation of perisylvian and calcarine anatomic landmarks within stereotaxic proportional coordinates. AJNR 1990;11:1123–1130.

26 Brierley JB, Beck E: The significance in human stereotactic brain surgery of individual variation in the diencephalon and globus pallidus. J Neurol Neurosurg Psychiatry 1959;22:287–298.
27 Berger M, Cohen W, Ojemann G: Correlation of motor cortex brain mapping data with magnetic resonance imaging. J Neurosurg 1990;72:383–387.
28 Ono M, Kubir S, Abernathey C: Atlas of the Cerebral Sulci. Stuttgart, Springer, 1990.
29 Pandya D, Rosene D: Some observations on trajectories and topography of commissural fibers; in Reeves J (ed): Epilepsy of the Corpus Callosum. New York, Plenum Press, 1985, pp 21–29.

R.M. Lehman, Department of Neurosurgery, Montreal Neurological Institute, Montreal, Que. (Canada)

Proceedings of the Meeting of the American Society for Stereotactic and Functional Neurosurgery, Pittsburgh, Pa., June 16–19, 1991
Stereotact Funct Neurosurg 1992;58:189–193

Comparison of CT- versus MRI-Guided, Computer-Assisted Depth Electrode Implantation

J.R. Smith[a], *T.L. Hardy*[b], *D.F. Rose*[c], *H.F. Flanigin*[a, d], *D.W. King*[d], *B.B. Gallagher*[d], *A.M. Murro*[d], *A. Fifer*[d]

[a] Section of Neurosurgery, and [d] Department of Neurology, Medical College of Georgia, Augusta, Ga.; [b] Department of Neurosurgery, Lovelace Medical Center, Albuquerque, N.M.; [c] Department of Neurology, VA Medical Center, Albuquerque, N.M., USA

Key Words. Depth electrodes · Image-guided, computer-assisted stereotactic implantation · Seizure focus localization · Magnetoencephalography

Abstract. Fourteen candidates for ablative seizure surgery underwent CT-guided, computer-assisted stereotactic depth electrode implantation and 21 underwent MRI-guided, computer-assisted implantation. A hand-held computer with no graphic capability was used for CT-guided procedures. A computer work station which included a high-resolution color graphics terminal with touchscreen interfacing and software capable of simulating targets and trajectories in single or multiple views was used for MRI-guided procedures. Previous phantom studies done with a 1.5-tesla MR scanner suggested acceptable localization error.

Localizing information was obtained in 10 (71.4%) of 14 of the CT-guided implants and in 16 (76.2%) of 21 of MRI-guided cases. In the CT group, 7 (70%) were seizure-free and 8 (80%) were >90% improved at 1 year follow-up. In the MRI group, 8 (80%) were seizure-free and 9 (90%) were >90% improved at latest follow-up.

Introduction

Stereotactic depth electrodes implanted with CT guidance without computer assistance will localize a seizure focus in approximately 70% of patients [1]. This may double the number of candidates for ablative seizure surgery [1] with a surgical outcome equivalent to that of patients undergoing surgery without invasive monitoring [2].

MRI provides enhanced visualization of neuroanatomic structures as well as multiplanar imaging capabilities. CT provides a lesser degree

1011–6125/92/0584–0189 $ 2.75/0

of anatomic resolution and does not allow target visualization in a second or third plane, which assists in defining the three-dimensional coordinates of a stereotactic target. This retrospective study was undertaken to analyze the localizing value of computer-assisted stereotactic depth electrode implantation under CT versus MRI guidance.

Methods and Materials

During 1989 and 1990, 14 patients underwent CT-guided depth electrode implantation into mesial temporal (MT) and extramesial temporal (XMT) areas. Target coordinates were derived with an HP41C computer and commercially available software (Radionics, Burlington, Mass., USA).

In 1990, 21 patients underwent MRI-guided stereotactic depth electrode implantation. Target coordinates and trajectories were derived using a commercially available computer work station with graphic rendering capabilities and touchscreen user interfacing (CASS-MIDCO, Albuquerque, N.M., USA) [3].

Depth electrode implantation was done on all patients with poor seizure localization on scalp-sphenoidal recordings, and on patients with localizing ictal recordings in whom significant divergent clinical, imaging or neuropsychologic data suggested a focus elsewhere [1]. All implants were done under local anesthesia and sedation. The Cosman-Roberts-Wells (CRW) stereotactic instrument was used in all cases. Eight-contact depth electrodes were used for all depth implants and monopolar electrodes were used for all epidural implants (PMT), Minneapolis, Minn., USA; AdTech, Racine, Wisc., USA).

Figure 1 shows two composite drawings of the implant types and trajectories. The majority of implants were of the type shown in the lower illustration. Occipitotemporal (OT) implants were used in most cases for monitoring of the MT region. Additional depth trajectories were used to monitor other limbic regions in selected cases. Stereotactically implanted epidural electrodes were used to monitor neocortical areas of interest. Vertex trajectories were used in 1 CT-guided and 3 MRI-guided cases to implant the hippocampus and in 2 CT-guided cases to implant the orbital frontal cortex [4]. Continuous video/EEG monitoring was carried out until at least 3–4 of the patient's habitual seizures had been recorded.

For CT-guided procedures, a GE 9800 CT scanner was used to obtain 1.5-mm slices at 3 mm intervals for target identification. Target coordinates obtained from the HP41C were transferred to the CRW apparatus. Avascular entry points were chosen after studying preimplant angiograms. A GE Signa 1.5-tesla unit was used for the MRI-guided procedures. T_1-weighted (TR 800, TE 20) sagittal 4-mm slices with 4.5 mm slice intervals and proton-density-weighted (TR 2000, TE 40) axial and coronal 3-mm slices with 3.5 mm slice intervals were obtained for target identification and trajectory simulation. These images were transferred from the MRI computer to the work station computer via a coaxial cable. Figure 2 shows an MRI multiplanar display of a simulated OT depth trajectory as seen on the computer work station monitor. After computer derivation of target coordinates, anteroposterior and lateral angles of trajectory are entered and displayed.

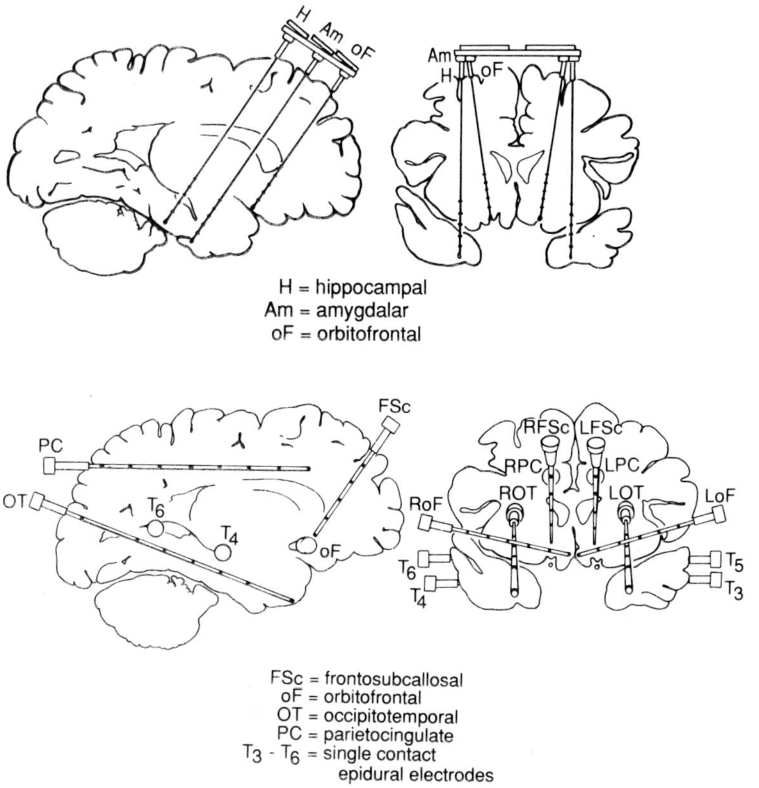

Fig. 1. Composite drawings of the implant types and trajectories.

Results

Localization was obtained in all MT implants, regardless of modality of image guidance. Localization was obtained in 7 of 11 (63.6%) CT-guided MT-XMT implants and in 9 of 14 (64.3%) MRI-guided MT-XMT implants (table 1). These results do not differ appreciably from our previous series of implants done with CT guidance but without computer assistance [1].

Ten patients from each group underwent surgery. In the CT group, 7 (70%) were seizure-free and 8 (80%) were >90% improved at 1 year follow-up. In the MRI group, 8 (80%) were seizure-free and 9 (90%) were >90% improved at most recent follow-up.

Table 1. Localization results: CT-versus MRI-guided depth electrode implants, 1989–1990

	MT localization	XMT localization	Non-localization
CT-guided			
MT (n = 3)	3		
MT-XMT (n = 11)	4	3	4
MRI-guided	7		
MT (n = 7)	7		
MT-XMT (n = 14	5	4	5

Complications

There was no permanent morbidity. There were 5 instances of transient global amnesia lasting from 5 to 30 min. All occurred during CT-guided left OT implants (fig. 1) in patients with ipsilateral verbal memory dominance confirmed by carotid amytal test.

One CT-guided MT-XMT case, which included OT implants, had non-localized seizure onsets. Postimplant radiographs suggested that both OT trajectories were immediately superior to the hippocampus. Subsequently placed vertex-entry hippocampal electrodes recorded bilateral independent seizures.

These observations suggest that implants guided by single-plane imaging without preimplant trajectory simulation may lead to complications or suboptimal localization.

Conclusions

Comparison of our results of seizure focus localization with CT versus MRI-guided depth electrodes revealed no significant difference. Similar surgical results occurred in both groups. This suggests an irreducible percentage of nonlocalizations and less than optimal surgical results. Review of our complications suggests that multiplanar imaging capability of MRI merged with computer graphic simulation may limit neurological complications and aid in seizure focus localization.

2 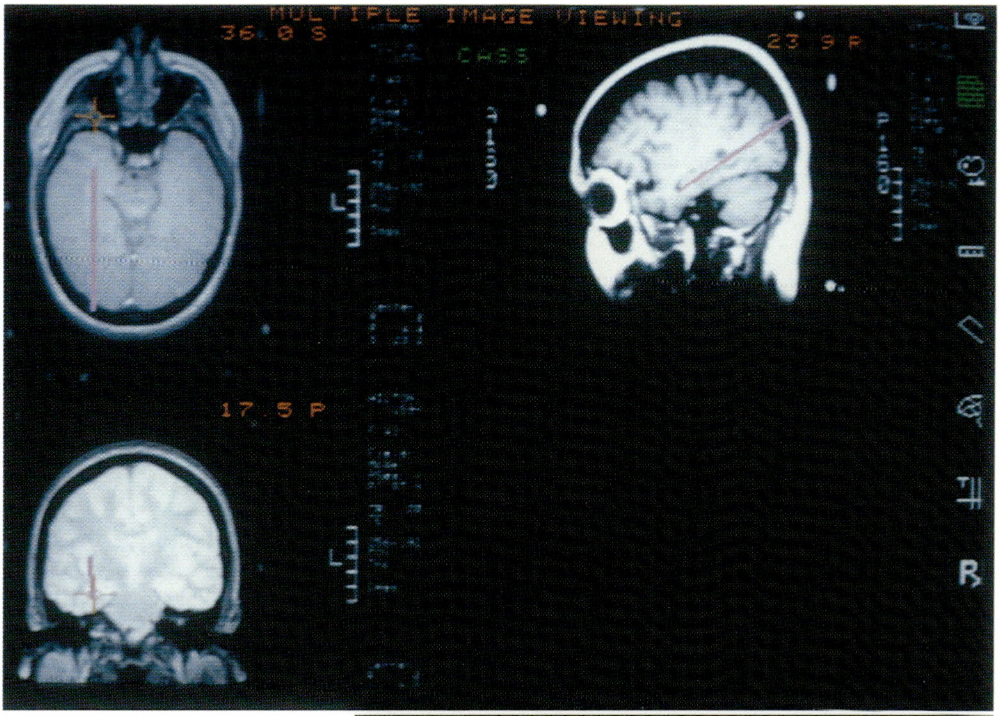

Fig. 2. MRI multiplanar display of a simulated OT depth electrode trajectory as seen on the computer work station monitor.

Fig. 3. Computer graphic rendering of an MEG-recorded magnetic dipole of an interictal epileptic discharge (maroon) superimposed on a CT scan using a common stereotactic reference plane. Wire frame rendering of the MEG sensors (red) is seen in the upper right corner.

3 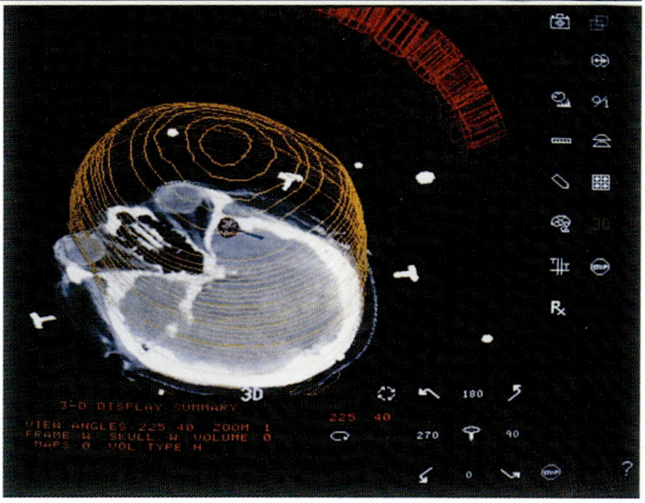

Addendum

Three-dimensional computer graphics merged with noninvasive functional imaging modalities such as magnetoencephalography (MEG) may in the future assist in localizing seizure foci not found with current invasive recording techniques. Presently, MEG provides spatial information on epileptic activity, but has limited accuracy [5, 6]. Development of more accurate mathematical methods may allow spatial characterization of multiple epileptic spikes in stereotactic space [7] and aid in seizure focus localization.

Figure 3 shows interictal epileptic activity recorded with a 37-channel MEG unit. These data were transferred to a computer work station and superimposed on a CT scan, using a common stereotactic reference plane.

References

1 Smith JR, Flanigin HF, King DW, et al: An 8-year experience with depth electrodes in the evaluation of ablative seizure surgery candidates. Stereotact Funct Neurosurg 1990;54/55:60–66.
2 Spencer SS: Depth electroencephalography in selection of refractory epilepsy patients for surgery. Ann Neurol 1981;9:207–214.
3 Hardy TL: Stereotactic CT atlases; in Lunsford LD (ed): Modern Stereotactic Neurosurgery. Boston, Nijhoff, 1988, pp 425–439.
4 Flanigin HF, Smith JR: Depth electrode implantation; in Engels J (ed): Surgical Treatment of the Epilepsies. New York, Raven Press, 1987, pp 609–612.
5 Barth DS, Sutherling W, Broffman J, Beatty J: Magnetic localization of a dipolar current source implanted in a sphere and a human cranium. EEG Clin Neurophysiol 1986;63:260–273.
6 Cohen D, Cuffin BN, Yunokuchi K, et al: MEG versus EEG localization test using implanted sources in the human brain. Ann Neurol 1990;28:811–817.
7 Rose DF: Magnetoencephalographs: Technology and equipment review. J Clin Neurophysiol 1991;8:238.

J.R. Smith, MD, Medical College of Georgia – Section of Neurosurgery,
1120 15th Street BIW-350B, Augusta, GA 30912-4010 (USA)

Proceedings of the Meeting of the American Society for Stereotactic and Functional Neurosurgery, Pittsburgh, Pa., June 16–19, 1991
Stereotact Funct Neurosurg 1992;58:194–199

Surgical Therapy of Temporal Lobe Seizures

Liu Zonghui, Tian Zengmin, Kang Guiquan, Cheng Li, Li Shiyue Chen Xiaohan, Fin Hanli, Zui Shihin

Department of Neurosurgery, Navy General Hospital of PLA, Beijing, China

Key Words. Epilepsy · Temporal lobe · Lesion resection

Abstract. Resection of epileptogenic lesions and pathological studies were performed in all 35 patients with temporal lobe epilepsy, 20 male and 15 female. Their ages ranged from 6 to 48 years with an average of 22 years. Various examinations including CT scan were carried out without any positive finding. EEG showed spike formation in the temporal lobes in all 35 patients. Epilepsy lesions were removed from the right temporal lobe in 22 patients and from the left temporal lobe in 13 patients. Pathological changes were found in all epilepsy lesions by light and electron microscopy. The operative outcomes were seizure-free since discharge in 10 patients (28.5%), seizure-free after some early attacks (34.2%) in 12 patients, seizure-free for 2 or more years and then rare or occasional attacks in 6 patients (17.1%), marked reduction of seizures in 5 patients (14.5%) and moderate or less reduction of seizure tendency in 2 patients (5.7%), with an effective rate of 93%. No death or severe complications did occur.

Epilepsy is not a single disease, but, rather is a constellation of symptoms or a syndrome. Drug treatment of the epilepsies, even when successful, is only suppressive, since none of the anticonvulsant drugs is curative and the cause of the seizures is not eliminated.

Operative efforts to bring relief for the patient with seizures undoubtedly date from very early times. Only during the last 5 decades, however, has an effective system of investigation and operative therapy been developed.

Epilepsy afflicts about 0.44% of the Chinese population. Of these cases, 25% are difficult to control with anticonvulsant medication and 10%, or about 450,000 individuals, are resistant to medical manage-

1011–6125/92/0584–0194 $ 2.75/0

ment. It is in this group that some patients are found to have focal brain damage as the cause of their seizures and can benefit from surgery.

In an attempt to elucidate the effect of treating temporal lobe seizures by operation, we performed an investigation of the clinical, EEG, social, psychological and pathological performance.

Clinical Material and Methods

35 patients with temporal lobe epilepsy were treated in the Navy General Hospital between January 1987 and January 1990. 20 patients were male and 15 female. Their ages ranged from 6 to 48 years, with an average of 22. The age at onset of seizures ranged from 1 to 27 years, with an average of 12. The etiology of the epilepsy was as follows: 5 patients suffered from birth trauma and 3 patients from encephalitis; 12 patients had a history of febrile seizures; 3 patients had familial epilepsy; 2 patients suffered from head trauma, and 10 patients had uncertain etiology.

All patients had been treated for years (mean = 13 years) and had taken all available medicine in monotherapeutic and polytherapeutic regimens. The types of epileptic attack were as follows: 12 cases of petit mal with grand mal; 10 cases of petit mal; 8 cases of grand mal; 5 cases of psychomotor attacks, and 10 cases of epileptic psychosis. The frequency of attacks was 10–20 times every day in 5 cases 1–10 times every day in 12 cases and 1–5 times every week in 15 cases; 12 cases had different levels of psychological symptoms. The 35 cases had no localizing symptoms on neurological examination. In all patients, the EEG disclosed the seizure spike activity in the temporal lobe. By the time of operation, most patients were severely handicapped and socially disabled by their seizures. The patients were all operated under general anesthesia through a lower temporal osteoplastic approach. Adequate exposure of the anterior and inferior portion of the temporal lobe is necessary for complete and safe removal of the inferior and medial parts of the lobe. After exposing the cortex, electrodes were placed on all parts of the temporal cortex. The activity was recorded while the anesthetic degree was adjusted to a level that resulted in the maximum amount of seizure activity. In some patients a depth electrode was also inserted to determine the origin of the spike as precisely as possible. Usually the spiking originated superficially, but in some cases spiking was also found in the depths of the temporal lobe. A small suction tip and coagulating forceps are used for the excision. It is very important to avoid careless manipulating and injuring the major vessels. The anterior temporal lobe was removed no further back than 4–6 cm to avoid postoperative dysphasia.

In this series, 22 cases involved removal of a focus of the right temporal lobe, and 13 cases had a focus of the left temporal lobe excised. During these operations, 10 cases underwent removal of the anterior temporal lobe and 10 cases of the temporal polar and mesiobasal region, including the hippocampus and amygdala, in 8 cases the temporal neocortical part and in cases the dorsolateral and laterobasal part were excised. If the removed area is limited, it is very useful to perform postexcision electrocorticography (ECoG) to detect any residual epileptic tissue. If it is safe to do so, such tissue is removed prior to closing the dura. The wound should be closed in multiple layers with a strict aseptic technique. Irrigation of tissues with a topical antibiotic solution and postoperative systemic antibiotics are recommended.

Results

Pathological Examination

The removed specimens of the 26 cases with temporal lobe epilepsy were examined by light and electron microscopy. In 19 cases the focal lesion was found and in 7 cases nonspecific changes were observed. Focal lesions included 4 cases of Ammon's horn sclerosis; 1 small abscess; 1 small astrocytoma; 1 small ganglioneuroma; 1 cicatrix lesion, and 11 cases of vascular lesions. The nonspecific changes (i.e. ultrastructural morphological changes) involved massive activation, in that preterminal synaptic vesicles were agglutinated, as well as increased dark neurocytes or morphological changes in neurons and walls of the capillaries.

Outcome of Operation

The cases were followed for 2–36 months (average 13 months). 10 cases were seizure-free since discharged (28.5%); 12 cases became seizure-free after some early attacks (34.2%); 6 cases were free for 2 or more years and then had rare or occasional attacks (17.1%); 5 cases showed marked reduction of seizure tendency (14.5%), and 2 cases had moderate or less reduction of seizure tendency (5.7%). There was no mortality, but 1 patient had hematoma opposite the operation site and 1 patient had wound infection.

Discussion

Further research on the function of the temporal lobe cortex [1–3] has revealed that the clinical manifestations and focus localization of temporal lobe epilepsy result from partial cerebral disease, and are not due to a specific cause as previously thought.

A temporal lobe seizure may consist of only a brief loss of orientation or a lack of consciousness, or the episode may last longer and be accompanied by automatic behavior [4–7]. The common signs of epileptic attacks are paresthesia in the upper abdomen, chest or throat, and phonism [5]. This seizure disorder is the commonest variety of epilepsy treated by the neurological surgeon. In about 50% of patients with temporal lobe epilepsy, Sommer's sector of Ammon's horn shows gliosis and loss of neurons.

In contrast to Penfield and Flanigin [2], who removed part of the temporal lobe to alleviate such seizures, temporal lobectomy, a resection that includes the medially placed amygdala and hippocampus [3–5], is now elected most frequently.

Falconer [5] emphasized the importance of asphyxia during infancy as a cause of mesial sclerosis; episodes of asphyxia occur in conjunction with status epilepticus, febrile convulsions, severe infection and head injury. In Falconer's [5] experience, the majority of subjects whose epilepsy was relieved by operation also showed markedly less aggressive behavior after the procedure. Penfield and Flanigin [2] reported on 60 cases of epilepsy, among which 20 cases had automatic behavior, 16 cases had epileptic psychosis or hallucinosis, 13 cases had asymmetry of movement and 5 cases had smell or chewing signs. Our 35 cases had no elevated cerebrospinal fluid pressure 16 cases had various signs, 9 had paresthesia in the chest and abdomen, 3 had phonism and photism, 2 had fright and 2 had hand washing and fumbling with clothes. Although these signs are helpful for the diagnosis of epilepsy, the localization of the focus must depend on EEG [8–13] with sphenoidal electrodes or 24-hour sleep deprivation EEG.

Pathological Changes in Epileptogenic Focus of Temporal Lobe

For further research of mechanisms, some scientists examine the removed focus pathologically based on ECoG. Penfield and Flanigin [2], after pathological study of the removed tissues, found atrophy, injury, abscess and scarring. Walsh and Delgada-Escueta [4] reported that, of 11 cases whose epileptogenic focus was examined, 8 cases had Ammon's horn sclerosis, 1 had an astrocytoma, 1 had an arteriovenous malformation (AVM) and another had diffuse gliosis. Rasmussen [1] reported that in 50% of epileptogenic foci of the temporal lobe the pathological change is cerebral scarring or degeneration of gliocytes, and 5% is small tumor or small AVM. Wieser and Yasargil [11] examined the removed amygdala and hippocampus of 23 cases with temporal lobe epilepsy and found 13 cases of tumor and 4 cases of Ammon's horn sclerosis. Bengaen reported that in a group of 35 cases there were

92% with abnormal change on pathological examination of epileptogenic foci of the temporal lobe, mainly gliosis and sclerosis.

Analysis of Treatment

Although the efficiency of removing the focus from the temporal lobe to treat epilepsy is confirmed, there are many factors influencing it. Heimburger et al. [9] think that it is necessary for attacking behavior of epilepsy to remove the temporal lobe. However, Walsh and Delgada-Escueta [4] reported an alleriation of only 20–40% of complicated and directed attack, which was due to the location of the focus in the frontal lobe of most of these patients. Bonis [10] reported that in 104 epileptic cases whose temporal lobes were removed the cure rate was 86.5%. In our group of 35 cases, epilepsy disappeared in 10 cases (28.5%) after operation, 12 cases were seizure-free after some early attacks (34.2%), and 6 cases were free for 2 or more years and then had rare or occasional attacks (17.1%), 5 cases had marked reduction of seizure tendency (14.5%) and 2 cases had moderate or less reduction of seizure tendency (5.7%), so generally 93% were improved.

To have a greater effect, ECoG examination should be performed again and again to look for the exact area of focus before operation and especially during operation, so that the focus can most thoroughly be removed under ECoG guidance. On pathological examination, the focus was abnormal in all 35 cases; this also showed that it is necessary to locate the focus exactly and remove the right area.

References

1 Rasmussen TH: Surgical aspects of temporal lobe epilepsy: Results and problems. Acta Neurochir Suppl 1980;30:1323.
2 Penfield W, Flanigin H: Surgical therapy of temporal lobe seizures. Arch Neurol Psychiatry 1950;64:491–500.
3 Wieser HG, Yasargil MG: Selective amygdalohippocampectomy as a surgical treatment of mesiobasal limbic epilepsy. Surg Neurol 1982;17:445–457.
4 Walsh GO, Delgada-Escueta AV: Complex partial seizures: Poor results of anterior temporal lobectomy. Neurology 1984;34:1–13.
5 Falconer MA: The significance of surgery for temporal lobe epilepsy in childhood and adolescence. J Neurosurg 1970;33:223–238.
6 Spencer DD, Spencer SS, et al: Access to the posterior medial temporal lobe structures in the surgical treatment of temporal lobe epilepsy. Neurosurgery 1984; 15:667–671.

7 Rausch R, Crandall PH: Psychological status related to surgical control of temporal lobe seizure. Epilepsia 1982;23:191–202.
8 Lieb JP, et al: Surface and deep EEG correlates of surgical outcome in temporal lobe epilepsy. Epilepsia 1982;23:1–13.
9 Heimburger RF, et al: Stereotaxic amygdalotomy for epilepsy with aggressive behavior. JAMA 1966;198:741–745.
10 Bonis A: Long-term results of cortical excisions based on stereotactic investigation in severe drug resistant epilepsies. Acta Neurochir Suppl 1980;30:55–66.
11 Wieser HG, Yasargil MG: Selective amygdalohippocampectomy as a surgical treatment of mesiobasal limbic epilepsy. Surg Neurol 1982;17:445–457.
12 Spencer DD, Spencer SS: Surgery of epilepsy. Neurol Clin 1985;3:313–330.
13 Olivier A, et al: The indications for and the role of depth electrode recording in epilepsy. Appl Neurophysiol 1983;46:33–36.

Liu Zonghui, Department of Neurosurgery, Navy General Hospital of PLA,
Beijing (China)

Proceedings of the Meeting of the American Society for Stereotactic and Functional Neurosurgery, Pittsburgh, Pa., June 16–19, 1991
Stereotact Funct Neurosurg 1992;58:200–208

Cerebellar Stimulation for Seizure Control: 17-Year Study

Ross Davis, Sandra E. Emmonds
Kennebec Valley Medical Center, Augusta, Me., USA

Key Words. Cerebellar stimulation · Seizures · Epilepsy · Behavior

Abstract. Since 1974, 32 seizure patients have undergone chronic cerebellar stimulation (CCS); 27 have been contacted with 9 (7 spastic, 2 epileptic) continuing to use CCS for an average of 14.3 years (10–17 years). 6 (67%) are seizure-free and 3 (33%) have a reduction of seizure frequency. In the last 2 years, 2 other patients with spastic seizures, who were using CCS for 13 years, died of respiratory illness; 1 had been seizure-free and the other had a reduction. Of the remaining 16 patients (12 spastic, 4 epileptic) who did use CCS for an average of 8.3 years (2–14 years) and now have nonfunctioning stimulators, 5 (31%) continue to be seizure-free, 7 (44%) have a reduction and 4 (25%) have no change or a slight increase. Overall, 23 (85%) patients have benefitted from CCS. Stimulation charge densities were 0.9–2.5 $\mu C/cm^2$/phase delivered at 10–180 pulses/sec to bilateral electrode pads on the superomedial cerebellar cortex. CCS is relatively safe and nonablative, and could be offered for patients with intractable seizures originating from bilateral or extratemporal foci.

The use of chronic cerebellar stimulation (CCS) as a therapy for intractable seizures in man was based on aminal studies from 1955, which were reviewed in 1980 by Laxer et al. [1], who found conflicting results. They drew two major conclusions; (1) stimulation of the vermis and intermediate cortex is more efficacious than stimulation of the lateral hemisphere, and (2) CCS is most effective in models of generalized or focal epilepsy of the limbic system, and least effective in models of focal epilepsy of the sensor imotor cortex.

Using CCS for the first time in epileptic patients in 1973, Cooper et al. [2, 3] later reported a reduction by at least 50% of the seizure activity in 18 of 34 patients. From 1977, 12 other clinical series, reviewed by

1011–6125/92/0584–0200 $ 2.75/0

Rossi et al. [4] and Davis and Emmons [5], reported on a further 95 seizure patients undergoing CCS. Of the total 129 seizure patients having CCS, 87 (67%) benefitted by seizure reduction. Thirty-two patients (27 with spastic seizures (SSP) and 5 with epileptic seizures (EP)) were ours and were reported in 1982–1984 [6, 7]; 19 (59%) were seizure-free, 8 (25%) had a reduction and 5 (16%) were not improved with CCS. In 1988, our follow-up report [5] on 28 (23 SSP, 5 EP) patients showed 16 (14 SSP, 2 EP) continuing to use CCS for an average of 11.1 years, with 12 (75%) seizure-free and 4 (25%) having a reduction. Of the 12 (9 SSP, 3 EP) cases no longer using CCS, 5 were seizure-free and 3 had reductions. The following report is an updated evaluation of our patients followed for the past 17 years.

Methods

Clinical Series

From February 1974, 331 spastic patients (89% with cerebral palsy) underwent CCS in our clinic [6] to reduce spasticity and improve function. However, 30 patients (9%) were having seizures during the 3 years prior to implantation and 6 EP patients underwent CCS specifically to reduce their intractable seizure activity [5–7].

CCS Equipment

From 1974 to 1978, we used the Avery Radiofrequency (RF) system (I-108 receiver, set at 0.5 mA, 0.5 ms, 180 pps, 7 min, alternating pulses; Avery Labs., Farmindale, N.Y., USA) with twin pad electrodes positioned bilaterally on the superomedial cerebellar surface. From May 1979, the SSP patients had a combination of the Avery electrodes connected with the totally implantable (TI) pulse generator Neurolith 601 (1.0–1.4 mA, 0.5 ms, 150 pps, 4 min, monodirectional pulses; Pacesetter Systems, Sylmar, Calif. USA). The charge density (QD = pulse current × width/electrode cathodal area) for both the Avery and Neurolith systems was in the range of 0.8–2.5 $\mu C/cm^2$/phase. The 5 EP patients had the Avery twin pad electrodes with a combination of different pulse generators (set at 10 pulses/s): Avery (RF) unit, Cordis (TI) Stimucor (Cordis, Miami, Fla., USA) and Neurodyne (TI) Epilith (table 1). Our surgical techniques and testing have been described in detail [5–7].

Results

Spastic Patients with Seizures

Of the 22 SSP patients reported in 1988 [5], 19 are described in table 1, of which 7 are still using stimulators while 12 are no longer using their external RF stimulators, or their internal TI units were depleted

Table 1. Cerebellar stimulation: detailed results of individual patients and their seizure and medication patterns

Name	DOB	Stimulator implanted[a]	CCS years	SSP ± Gen. pre.	SSP ± Gen. 1991
SSP patients with functioning CCS					
MB	4/3/68	76 A→91 N	15		
RE	10/11/59	77 A	14		
JHa	11/13/50	76 A	15		
SH	9/23/69	76 A→88 N	15		
JJ	10/1/67	77 A→88 N	14		
BP	11/30/71	81 N→91 N	10	1/2w	F
BS	11/25/64	77 A	14	1–3/m	F
KB[b]	6/1/64	76 A→89 N	13		
JHo[b]	4/1/69	77 A→88 N	12		
Results: seizure-free = 5; reduced = 2; patient SH: CP ± same; patients KB and JHo: died 1989, 1 seizure-free, 1 reduced					
SSP patients with nonfunctioning CCS					
TB	1/12/71	1/76 A	13		
DB	10/20/60	1/75 A	12		
CF	2/25/76	3/81 N	9		
LH	1/19/59	12/76 A	13		
CK	4/9/67	9/76 A	13		
CL[c]	8/13/65	3/76 A	5	1–2/m	F
DM[c]	3/56	78 A	8		
BM	10/1/70	79 N	4		
JS	2/3/67	8/78 A	5		
PS[c]	6/8/57	5/75 A	6		
DC[b]	7/72	77 A	2		
RC[b]	10/75	79 N	6		
Results: seizure-free = 5; reduced = 4; no change = 1; increased = 2					
EP patients with functioning CCS					
BC	7/61	76 C→81 C	15		
JG	58	74 A→90 C	17		
Results: seizure-free = 1; reduced = 1					
EP patients with nonfunctioning CCS					
CB	72	77 A	2	30/d	1+/d
LL	9/54	75 A→80 C	14		

CP ± Gen.		Gen. T/C		Gen. abs.		Gen. myo.		Medications	
pre.	1991	pre.	1991	pre.	1991	pre.	1991	pre.	1991
12/y	10/y							2	3
1/y	F							0	0
1–2/w	F							1	0
10/d	same	4/m	F					2	1
50+/d	1–2/d							2	4
								2	1
								1	1
2–10/d	2/y							2	1
1–3/w	F							0	0
1/y	F							2	1
						75/d	3/y	2	1
				2/m	F			3	1
		1–5/y	2/m					2	1
2–3/w	3/m							2	1
								2	0
1–5/m	F							3	2
1/w	1/d							2	1
2/y	1–2/y							1	1
1/2–3y	F							3	1
						1–2/m	1/3y	1	0
10/d	5/d							4	5
				50+/d	F			4	4
20/d	1/m								
								4	3
				15–25/d	3/m			2	3

Table 1 (continued)

Name	DOB	Stimulator implanted[a]	CCS years	SSP ± Gen. pre.	SSP ± Gen. 1991
RL	7/67	79 C	8		
JM	3/60	80 E→83 C	3		

Results: seizure-free = 0; reduced; = 3; no change = 1

DOB = Date of birth (month/day/year); Gen. = generalized; CP = cerebral palsy; T/C = tonic/clonic; abs. = absences; myo. = myoclonus; pre. = before stimulation; y = year; F = seizure-free; w = week; d = day; m = month.
[a] Year or month/year of implantation and type of stimulator: A = Avery; N = Neurolith; C = cordis; E = epilith.
[b] 1989 data.
[c] 1990 data.

or removed. In the last 2 years, 2 other SSP patients (KB, JHo) who were using CCS for 13 years died of respiratory illness; 1 had been seizure-free and the other had a reduction.

Of the 7 patients using CCS for an average time of 13.6 years (10–15 years), 5 (71%) are seizure-free and 2 (29%) have a reduction of seizure frequency. Of the 12 SSP patients who used CCS for an average of 8 years (range: 2–13) but have ceased with stimulation for an average of 5.9 years (range: 1–12), 5 (42%) have remained free of seizures, 4 (33%) are reduced and 3 (25%) have returned to prestimulation levels or have slight increases (table 1). Seizure medication numbers are listed in table 1; 17 (65%) needed less medication, 5 (19%) had no increase and 4 (15%) needed increases.

Epilepsy per se

Of the 6 patients who underwent CCS for intractable epilepsy from 1974, 5 were described and evaluated in 1982–1984 [6–7], and again in 1988 [5], and are updated in table 1. Patient JG was added, as she underwent bilateral Avery RF receiver replacements with a Cordis Stimucor TI unit by ourselves in February 1990. Her original system was im-

CP ± Gen.		Gen. T/C		Gen. abs.		Gen. myo.		Medications	
pre.	1991	pre.	1991	pre.	1991	pre.	1991	pre.	1991
50+/d	same							4	3
5/d	1/d					50+/d	F	6	3

planted by Dr. I.S. Cooper in 1974 for her complex-partial epilepsy with generalized seizures (20/day); she has been followed by Dr. R.S. Dow (Portland, Oreg., USA) who now reports that although she has one to several minor seizures at the time of her menses, she has been able to increase her work output at the sheltered workshop from 95 cents/h (1989) to US $2.95/h (1990–1991). Her interictal spike frequencies were recorded and computer-analyzed by Zeng et al. [8]. When CCS was on, 44 paroxysmal epileptiform discharges (PDs) wree recorded in 73 min of random samples; however, 119 PDs were recorded in similar sampling with the CCS off. Upton [9], in 1978, reported significant reductions in PDs in 3 other EP patients during and after CCS.

Patient BC has used CCS for 15 years and is seizure-free of his generalized absences (50/day in 1976) with behavioral improvements enabling him to work. Of the 4 no longer using stimulation, patient RL who used CCS for 8 years did have sustained benefits of reduced seizures and improved functioning. When the battery depleted she regressed and was placed in a nursing home awaiting finances for a replacement. Patient LL had 14 years of CCS where her 15–25/day absences with generalized seizures have been reduced to 2/month, which is sustained after the battery depleted 2 years ago, whereas the other 2 cases (CB, JM) with only 2 and 3 years of CCS have continued to have fewer seizures.

Patients CK and JM had an infection of the tissues around their stimulator, which were removed with recovery. Otherwise there have been no other patient complications.

Discussion

Stimulation has not caused any aggravation of the seizure conditions, nor any deterioration in patients' neurological disabilities during the years of CCS [4, 5]. The study has certainly indicated that CCS at the charge densities (QD: 1–2.5 $\mu C/cm^2$/phase) has not initiated seizures. The wide range of stimulation frequencies (10–180 pps) and sequencing used in our series did not appear to be a factor in the seizure control by CCS. We do recommend 10 pps with a 4-min on/off sequencing. The use of the TI units has been a major factor in the safety and success in controlling the seizure patients, particularly those with behavioral problems, because the units cannot be damaged or setting changed by the patients or families.

D. Goldman and R.S. Dow [pers. commun.] have reviewed the statistical data of Van Buren et al.'s [10] double-blind study of 5 EP patients undergoing CCS, and found contrary evidence to the published conclusions of 'no significant difference'. After correcting their percentage change equation to read [(postoperative frequency – preoperative frequency)/preoperative frequency] $\times 100\%$, and then converting the percentage changes in their table 2 to seizures/day, they found that, although 3 of the 5 patients had an increase in their seizure counts after the implantation without stimulation, nevertheless the first 4 patients showed decreased seizure rates by 73, 69, 73 and 85%, respectively, during the CCS on phases compared to the off periods of their double-blind study. We also have recalculated the results from their table 2 [10] and confirm that the first 4 patients of their 5 had reduced seizures/day with CCS in their double-blind study. We also note in their report [10] that their family evaluations indicated 'increased alertness, interest in surroundings, and diminished intra-family strife were most frequently cited. The seizures seemed less severe, of shorter duration, and less debilitating'. Realistically, the 1978 Van Buren et al.'s [10] report had a negative effect on the further use of CCS for intractable seizure control, even though 11 of 12 other clinics [4, 5] published reports showing seizure reductions in 87 (75%) of 115 seizuring patients with cerebellar stimulation.

Overall, of our 27 patients re-evaluated, 23 (85%) have benefitted from the long-term use of CCS, all 11 patients using CCS are benefitting, with a definite carry-over or cumulative effect in 12 (75%) of the 16 not continuing to use CCS. This carry-over effect was observed by Bidzinski et al. [11] in 4 of 12 EP patients undergoing only 10–12 days of stimulation with temporary leads. One year later, they reported the 4 cases as still significantly improved. The above results from CCS do compare favorably with the 62% effective results (43% seizure-free, 20% reduction) obtained from cerebral cortical resection in 58 children followed for 1–14 years, who had undergone preoperative epidural recording arrays and found to have epilepsy of non-neoplastic, extratemporal origin, as reported in 1987 by Goldring [12].

Conclusion

The evidence is that CCS is efficacious and that implantation is a relatively safe (nonablative, noninvasive) procedure to offer patients with medically intractable epilepsy originating from bilateral or extratemporal foci. A TI stimulator is a necessity, set at a QD of 1–2.5 $\mu C/cm^2$/phase. Electrode pads should be small in thickness and width, with a protective posterior pad, and positioned on the superomedial cerebellar cortical surface so stimulation is symmetrical and synchronous. Regular testing of equipment and medication adjustments are necessary.

References

1 Laxer KD, Robertson LT, Julien RM, et al: Phenytoin: Relationship between cerebellar function and epileptic discharges; in Glaser GH, Penry J, Woodbury DM (eds): Antiepileptic Drugs: Mechanism of Action. New York, Raven Press, 1980, pp 415–427.

2 Cooper IS, Amin I, Riklan M, et al: Chronic cerebellar stimulation in epilepsy: Clinical and anatomical studies. Arch Neurol 1976;33:559–570.

3 Cooper IS, Ricklan M, Amin I, et al: A long-term follow-up study of cerebellar

stimulation for the control of epilepsy; in Cooper IS (ed): Cerebellar Stimulation in Man. New York, Raven Press, 1978, pp 19–38.
4 Rossi GF, Colicchio G, Scerrati M: La stimolazione cerebellare cronica nel trattamento dell'epilessia farmacoresistente, Boll Lega Ital Epil 1987;60:5–12.
5 Davis R, Emmons SE: Safety and efficacy of cerebellar stimulation for seizure control. Boll Lega Ital Epil 1988;64:105–115.
6 Davis R, Engle H, Kudzma J, et al: Update of chronic cerebellar stimulation for spasticity and epilepsy. Appl Neurophysiol 1982;45:44–50.
7 Davis R, Gray E, Engle H, et al: The reduction of seizures in cerebral palsy and epileptic patients using chronic cerebellar stimulation; in Davis R, Bloedel JR (eds): Cerebellar Stimulation for Spasticity and Seizures. Boca Raton, CRC Press, 1984, pp 247–261.
8 Zeng J, Smith DB, DeToledo J, Dow RS: The effect of cerebellar stimulation on interictal spike frequency. Abstr 1990 Am Epil Soc Mett Epilepsia, in press.
9 Upton ARM: Neurophysiological mechanisms in modification of seizures; in Cooper IS (ed): Cerebellar Stimulation in Man. New York, Raven Press, 1978, pp 39–57.
10 Van Buren JM, Wood JH, Oakley J, et al: Preliminary evaluation of cerebellar stimulation by double-blind and stimulation and biological criteria in the treatment of epilepsy. J Neurosurg 1978;48:407–416.
11 Bidzinski J, Bacia T, Ostrowski K, et al: Effect of cerebellar cortex electrostimulation on the frequency of seizures in drug-resistant epilepsy. Neurol Neurochir Pol 1981;31:605–609.
12 Goldring S: Surgical management of epilepsy in children; in Engel J (ed): Surgical Treatment of the Epilepsies. New York, Raven Press, 1987, pp 445–464.

Ross Davis, Section of Neurosurgery, Kennebec Valley Medical Center, Augusta, ME 04330 (USA)

Announcements

World Society for Stereotactic and Functional Neurosurgery

Plans are being finalized to hold the 1993 meeting of the World Society for Stereotactic and Functional Neurosurgery in beautiful Ixtapa, Mexico, October 11th–15th, 1993. This extraordinary Pacific resort will be a wonderful venue for the WSSFN meeting, which will be held immediately before the October, 1993 meeting of the World Federation of Neurosurgical Societies in Acapulco, Mexico.

For additional information, please contact:
Philip L. Gildenberg, M.D., Ph.D.
6560 Fannin – Suite 1530
Houston, Texas 77030
Phone: 713-790-0795
Fax: 713-669-0388

The Medtronic Award in Functional Neurosurgery

The World Society for Stereotactic and Functional Neurosurgery is pleased to announce that Medtronic, Inc., will sponsor 'The Medtronic Award in Functional Neurosurgery', to be conferred on the occasion of the XIth Meeting in Ixtapa, Mexico. As part of Medtronic's continuing commitment to post graduate education and to advancing the state of knowledge in various areas of the medical field, including a strong commitment to encourage young neurosurgeons to develop an interest in functional neurosurgery, the company will bestow an honorarium of as $ 500, in addition to business class travel and hotel costs to attend the meeting, and a per diem allowance for other meeting expenses.

The Medtronic Award in Functional Neurosurgery is intended to encourage young neurosurgeons or neuroscientists to develop an interest in functional neurosurgery and is limited to individuals doing investigations in this field as it relates to nervous system function and/or how activation of the system by electricity or by chemical infusion can alter or improve function. Preference in selection will be given to individuals in the early stages of their careers, i.e., those who have not yet completed their neurosurgery or neuroscience training or have done so within the previous 10 years.

Selection will be based on a full manuscript submitted to the Awards Committee at the time of abstract submission for the XIth World Society for Stereotactic and Functional Neurosurgery Meeting. The deadline is May 15, 1993. The winner will present his or her work at a special 'Medtronic Young Scientist Lecture during the meeting.

Further details will be included in the meeting literature.

The Elekta Radionics/Trent Wells Award in Stereotactic Neurosurgery

Through the generosity of Elekta Instruments AB and Radionics, Inc., The World Society for Stereotactic and Functional Neurosurgery is pleased to announce that 'The Elekta/Radionics/Trent Wells Award in Stereotactic Neurosurgery' will again be awarded at the XIth Meeting in Ixtapa, Mexico.

The 'The Elekta/Radionics/Trent Wells Award in Stereotactic Neurosurgery' has been created to encourage advances in neuroscience through imaginative use of stereotaxis and is open to residents, graduate students, or individuals who have been in practice less than 10 years. Candidates need not be neurosurgeons, but should be potential members of the World Society for Stereotactic and Functional Neurosurgery or one of the regional societies.

The award will include an honorarium of US $ 500 and all travel and support costs for the winner to attend the meeting. The winner will be specially recognized and will present his or her work at the scientific meeting. The award will be made for the best eligible presentation submitted to the World Society for Stereotactic and Functional Neurosurgery Program Committee on a subject related to stereotactic neurosurgery. Applicants should indicate that they wish their work to be considered for the 'The Elekta/Radionics/Trent Wells Award in Stereotactic Neurosurgery' in the appropriate place on the official abstract form.

Author Index

Subject Index